THE CHINA STUDY

QUICK & EASY COOKBOOK

COOK ONCE, EAT ALL WEEK WITH
WHOLE FOOD, PLANT-BASED RECIPES

DEL SROUFE

EDITED BY LEANNE CAMPBELL, PhD | FOREWORD BY THOMAS M. CAMPBELL, MD

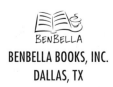

BenBella

BENBELLA BOOKS, INC.
DALLAS, TX

Recipes are based on the research of T. Colin Campbell as presented in *The China Study* (BenBella Books, 2005), coauthored by T. Colin Campbell, PhD, & Thomas M. Campbell, MD.

BenBella Books, Inc.
10300 N. Central Expressway
Suite #530
Dallas, TX 75231
www.benbellabooks.com
Send feedback to feedback@benbellabooks.com

Printed in the United States of America
10 9 8 7 6 5 4 3 2 1

Library of Congress Cataloging-in-Publication Data
Sroufe, Del, author.
    The China study quick & easy cookbook : cook once, eat all week with whole food, plant-based recipes / Del Sroufe ; edited by LeAnne Campbell, PhD ; foreword by Tom Campbell.
        pages   cm
    Includes bibliographical references and index.
    ISBN 978-1-940363-81-3 (paperback) — ISBN 978-1-940363-91-2 (electronic)
    1. Vegetarian cooking.   2. Cooking (Vegetables)   3. Quick and easy cooking   I. Campbell, LeAnne, editor.   II. Title.
    TX837.S7165   2015
    641.5'12—dc23   2014037775

Editing by LeAnne Campbell
Copyediting by Shannon Kelly
Proofreading by Laura Cherkas, Clarissa Phillips, and Greg Teague
Indexing by JigSaw Indexing
Front cover by Bradford Foltz
Full cover by Sarah Dombrowsky
Photography by Robert Metzger
Food styling by Steven Thomas
Text design by Kit Sweeney
Text composition by Aaron Edmiston
Printed by Versa Press, Inc.

Distributed by Perseus Distribution
www.perseusdistribution.com

To place orders through Perseus Distribution:
Tel: 800-343-4499
Fax: 800-351-5073
E-mail: orderentry@perseusbooks.com

Significant discounts for bulk sales are available. Please contact Glenn Yeffeth at glenn@benbellabooks.com or 214-750-3628.

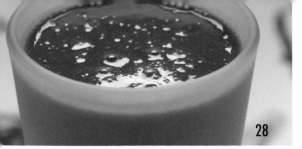

28

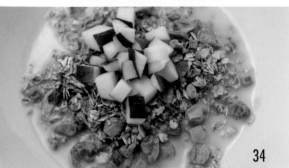

34

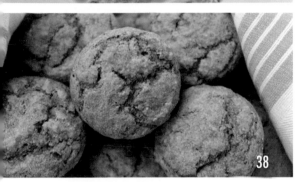

38

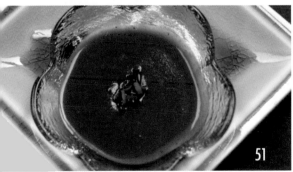

51

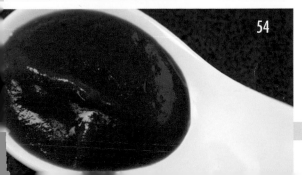

54

CONTENTS

RECIPES

BREAKFAST DISHES

SAUCES, SALAD DRESSINGS & SEASONINGS

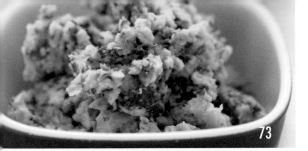
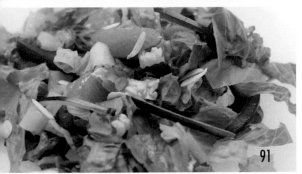
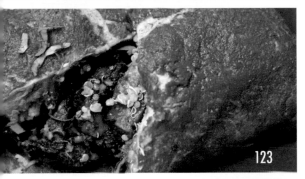
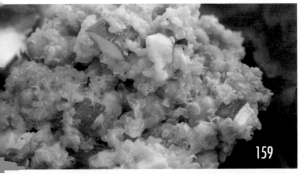
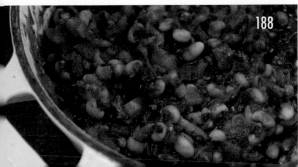

SOUPS

ENTRÉES

DESSERTS

APPENDIX

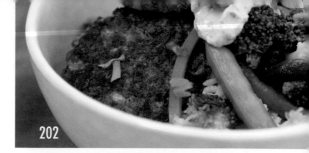

202

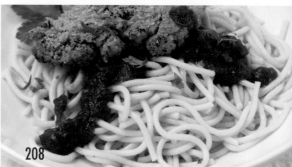

208

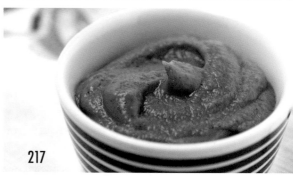

217

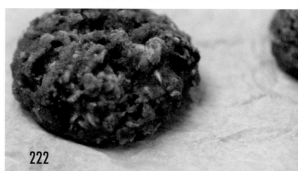

222

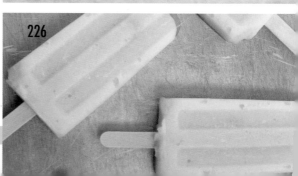

226

FOREWORD

When we published *The China Study* hardcover edition at the beginning of 2005, neither my dad nor I had high expectations. We had a hard time getting the manuscript published, having been told that the book needed to be at least 50 percent recipes and menu plans. It was even suggested that we come up with a different diet for each of the different disease conditions we discuss in order to create something more catchy and enticing for the readers. In the end, we were fortunate to find an independently thinking partner in BenBella Books, a publisher in Texas, far from the big publishing houses who seemed confined to formulas and supposedly sure things.

Looking back at that difficult start ten years ago, it is with enormous gratitude that I introduce the third China Study cookbook. I am grateful for all the readers who have shared their stories and comments about how *The China Study* has contributed to their own personal health and healing. It turns out that people want intelligent, science-based information to improve their lives; not just to live longer but to improve their health and happiness in the near term as well. This is what a healthy diet and lifestyle can do. Making the best choices for food, drink, and physical activity collectively is far more powerful than anything else you might consider for long-term health.

Now, as a practicing family physician, I spend many patient encounters working to help people take control of their health, partly by communicating the scientific rationale for a whole food, plant-based diet. And as the director of the T. Colin Campbell Center for Nutrition Studies, I continue to encourage scientific understanding of the optimal diet. But while the science is thought provoking and convincing, the practical application of a whole food, plant-based diet is equally important. When we wrote *The China Study*, we wanted to fully elaborate on the scientific and socioeconomic factors surrounding optimal nutrition and did not feel we could do justice to the practical information in the same book. We resisted those early attempts to include recipes and menu plans, knowing that other people could cover these aspects of dietary practice far better than we could.

Chef Del is just such a person. Del is one of a small handful of chefs in America who has moved beyond oils and processed foods to offer health-promoting recipes that remain tasty, convenient, and easy. He has intimate personal experience with poor health while consuming a vegan diet rich in processed foods, and he successfully overcame his personal challenges to regain his health by shifting to a more whole food, plant-based diet. He has been cooking healthy food for people day after day for many years as part of wellness programs and created the wonderful recipe collections found in *Better Than Vegan* and *Forks Over Knives: The Cookbook*.

Chef Del's recipes in this third China Study cookbook are particularly useful for highlighting the ease and convenience of eating an optimal diet. Very few people have the time and desire to cook food all day. We need something fast that doesn't sacrifice taste or health. In our toxic food environment comprised of grocery stores that greet you with walls of sugar cereal and giant bins of candy, food that is fast, tasty, and healthy almost seems to be a highly elusive, nearly mystical goal. But with the book you now hold in your hands, it is entirely achievable.

Once you appreciate the power of a whole food, plant-based diet, it is easy to think of chefs who pave the way toward healthier eating as true healers. Given his impressive resume, Chef Del has been a master healer for many years now, and it is my hope that his recipes in this book will pave the way to new health for you and your family. There is perhaps no more powerful "how-to" diet book than a good cookbook like this one. Enjoy, be well, and good luck!

—THOMAS M. CAMPBELL II, MD
Coauthor of *The China Study*
Author of *The Campbell Plan*

INTRODUCTION

When I was a kid, my mother, a divorced working parent, always managed to get dinner on the table. Working a full-time job meant that she was out of the house by 7:00 a.m. and did not get home until almost 6:00 p.m. every night. To put dinner on the table at a decent hour, she had to have a plan. Sometimes that plan meant that she would make quick, easy-to-prepare meals like hamburgers or Polish sausage with peppers and onions. Often she would be preparing two meals at once—a quick and easy dish for that night and something more complicated, like a turkey roast, for the next few nights. She was a master at taking one dish and using it in a variety of ways so that we were not eating leftovers all the time. For example, that roasted turkey would be eaten freshly cooked with sautéed vegetables and rice, and then the next night the leftovers would be used to make turkey à la king. Unbaked meatloaf was often divided in two: part of it would be baked as meatloaf and the rest made into spaghetti and meatballs. Between all these amazing meals, I thought my mom had magic powers, and I wanted to have those same powers. So I started cooking and doing what Mom did.

When I opened my commercial kitchen at Wellness Forum Foods with my business partner Pam Popper in 2006 to serve as the home of my plant-based meal delivery service, catering kitchen, and manufacturing hub for the wide variety of products sold at the Wellness Forum, I used the same principles to make my menu interesting.

Our Maple-Ginger Baked Tofu is used to make three or four different kinds of wraps as well as our Zen Bowl and occasionally even sloppy joes. My favorite oven-fried tofu recipe is sold as is, with barbecue sauce, and then often added to several specials we make on a regular basis, such as Tofu Cacciatore, Tofu Creole, and enchiladas.

This philosophy of multi-purposing recipes is in part what motivated me to write this cookbook. As I work to take charge of my own health, I want whole, low-fat, plant-based food on my dinner table. While I enjoy creating (and eating) more elaborate recipes, I also come home at night and want a healthy dinner in a hurry. And though times are changing, I still can't call up any of my local restaurants and get an oil-free stir-fry delivered to my house.

My basic plan for feeding myself is simple. On Saturdays I determine what I want to eat the following week. Sometimes I keep a running list of dishes I want to try or foods that I am craving. I also look at my calendar to see how many meals I will need for the week. There's no point in cooking for twenty-one meals when I will only be available for fourteen of them. I also usually leave the weekends open for eating out or enjoying leftovers.

So, after all my considerations, I decide what I want to make and how I will use it. Almost everything I make gets used in at least two different dishes. For example, peanut sauce goes on Thai pizza and in a rice and veggie wrap. Brown rice is a staple used in many dishes from break-fast to a late-night snack. Once I have the weekly menu finalized, I check to make sure that I have everything I need in my pantry. Keeping my pantry fully stocked means I don't have to make unexpected and unplanned trips to the store. If I am missing a particular ingredient, I add it to my shopping list to make one convenient trip.

Finally, with my menu planned and my ingredients ready, I look at the recipes to see how much I'll cook ahead of time and what will get finished during the week. For example, stir-fry sauce gets prepared on Sunday but won't be used in a stir-fry until the night I plan to eat it. This is a good way of making meal preparations easy throughout the week, so I recommend that you try similar methods if, like me, you want to eat healthfully without sacrificing time or variety.

To adopt my "cook once, eat all week" strategy in your kitchen, I suggest that you make a similar plan to the one I mentioned above. Take a look at the recipes in this cookbook. They are a combination of dishes that are easy to prepare and that can be used in many ways. These are the recipes that keep me on track as I pursue my plant-based healthy lifestyle, while also allowing me to enjoy delicious food that isn't a challenge to prepare.

You can prepare most of them in less than thirty minutes. Many basic recipes are also used in multiple dishes throughout the book, and once you have familiarized yourself with them and tried a few out, you may even have a few ideas of your own about how to use some of these recipes in *your* favorite dishes.

Once you decide upon the recipes you'd like to cook, you can start mapping out your menu for the week. Create a shopping list and double-check your pantry to make sure you have everything you need to prepare the dishes you have chosen. This way, you'll only go to the store once and not three or four times—which I have done when I was not prepared. For your convenience, all of the sample menu plans I've provided include a shopping list of additional food items for each week, and there is also a general pantry list to help you stock all of the ingredients you need to make the recipes in this book.

Everything you need to eat healthfully without spending all day, every day in the kitchen is here in your grasp. I hope you'll find that cooking this way makes life easier—and makes healthy eating fun.

—CHEF DEL

SAMPLE MENU PLANS

MENU PLAN I

This menu plan is for the household of one or two that doesn't mind leftovers. It is perfect in the summer when basil is fresh from the garden and corn is fresh from the field.

Most of these recipes make four servings. Keep fresh mixed greens on hand for salads and have your favorite toppings ready to add to your salad throughout the week. For this menu, you will need the recipes listed below, as well as the items in the additional ingredients list. See the pantry list on p. 21 for items you should always have on hand.

MAKE IT EASY: Make your salad in a large bowl at the beginning of the week and add your salad dressing to serve.

MENU		ADDITIONAL INGREDIENTS
Tomato, Corn, and Fresh		2 bananas
Basil Soup	163	2 or 3 large apples
Southwest Burgers	125	4½ cups fresh basil
All-Purpose Vinaigrette (×2)	44	4 large tomatoes
Basil Pesto Hummus	73	1 small jar salsa
Falafel Tacos	205	3 ripe avocados
Falafel	82	4 red onions
Green Sauce	52	1 small bunch green onions
Apple Pie Granola	34	1 lemon
Penne with Fresh Herbed Tomato-		1 small bunch fresh parsley
Corn Salsa	136	1 large bunch fresh cilantro
Fresh Herbed Tomato-		1 jalapeño pepper
Corn Salsa (×2)	58	1 cucumber
Tostadas	207	1 pint cherry tomatoes
		1½ cups alfalfa sprouts
		1 pound mixed greens
		1 head romaine lettuce

MONDAY

BREAKFAST
Apple Pie Granola with
    fresh chopped apples and
    unsweetened nondairy
    milk

LUNCH
Tomato, Corn, and Fresh
    Basil Soup
mixed greens salad with
    cherry tomatoes, cucumber
    slices, red onion slices, and
    garbanzo beans (chick-
    peas) with All-Purpose
    Vinaigrette

DINNER
Southwest Burgers
mixed greens salad with
    cherry tomatoes, cucum-
    ber slices, red onion slices,
    and garbanzo beans with
    All-Purpose Vinaigrette

TUESDAY

BREAKFAST
Apple Pie Granola with
    fresh chopped apples and
    unsweetened nondairy
    milk

LUNCH
leftover Southwest Burgers
mixed greens salad with
    cherry tomatoes, cucum-
    ber slices, red onion slices,
    and garbanzo beans with
    All-Purpose Vinaigrette

DINNER
Falafel Tacos
mixed greens salad with
    cherry tomatoes, cucum-
    ber slices, red onion slices,
    and garbanzo beans with
    All-Purpose Vinaigrette

WEDNESDAY

BREAKFAST
Apple Pie Granola with
    banana slices, chopped
    dates, and unsweetened
    nondairy milk

LUNCH
Basil Pesto Hummus wrap
    with alfalfa sprouts and
    sliced cucumber
mixed greens salad with
    cherry tomatoes, cucum-
    ber slices, red onion slices,
    and garbanzo beans with
    All-Purpose Vinaigrette

DINNER
Tostadas
mixed greens salad with
    cherry tomatoes, cucum-
    ber slices, red onion slices,
    and garbanzo beans with
    All-Purpose Vinaigrette

BREAKFAST
Apple Pie Granola with banana slices, chopped dates, and unsweetened nondairy milk

LUNCH
leftover Tomato, Corn, and Fresh Basil Soup

mixed greens salad with cherry tomatoes, cucumber slices, red onion slices, and garbanzo beans with All-Purpose Vinaigrette

DINNER
Penne with Fresh Herbed Tomato-Corn Salsa

mixed greens salad with cherry tomatoes, cucumber slices, red onion slices, and garbanzo beans with All-Purpose Vinaigrette

BREAKFAST
Apple Pie Granola with fresh chopped apples, chopped dates, and unsweetened nondairy milk

LUNCH
leftover Penne with Fresh Herbed Tomato-Corn Salsa

DINNER
Falafel Tacos

mixed greens salad with cherry tomatoes, cucumber slices, red onion slices, and garbanzo beans with All-Purpose Vinaigrette

MENU PLAN II

The key to saving time in cooking is to cross-purpose some basics like Almost Instant Peanut Sauce or Mushrooms Barbacoa and use them in different recipes to give you variety without a lot of effort. Making double batches of dishes and then using them in a variety of ways is one way around eating too many leftovers in a week.

I like to cook a big pot of quinoa or brown rice once a week to use in recipes throughout the week and to have as last-minute side dishes or stir-fries. Cooked grains like rice or quinoa make the easiest meals. Sometimes I eat brown rice warmed with almond milk, a dash of cinnamon, and dried fruit like raisins or dates as a quick breakfast. I also make Date and Soy Stir-Fry Sauce every week so I can make stir-fry with rice and vegetables as a last-minute meal.

I make one or two salad dressings at the beginning of the week and keep fresh salad greens on hand, so I can always have healthy salad options. I also keep my favorite salad vegetables on hand—cherry tomatoes, garbanzo beans, raisins, sliced green onion, and so on.

For this menu, you will need the recipes listed below, as well as the items in the additional ingredients list. See the pantry list on p. 21 for items you should always have on hand.

MAKE IT EASY: On Sunday, put together all the components for recipes like the Mushroom Tacos, the barbacoas, and the burritos and then assemble them as needed throughout the week so that you can enjoy them fresh.

MENU		ADDITIONAL INGREDIENTS
Asian Noodle Soup (×2)	166	nondairy milk
Beans and Grain Salad	103	fresh fruit
White Bean–Miso Spread (×2)	77	4½ pounds portobello mushrooms
Pasta with Vegetables and		6 cups slaw mix
White Bean–Miso Spread (×2)	144	4 bunches fresh spinach (about 16 cups)
Portobello Mushroom Burgers	124	1 small head Chinese cabbage
Fresh Spinach Salad (×2)	88	1 8-ounce package shiitake mushrooms
All-Purpose Vinaigrette	44	2 red bell peppers
Mushroom Tacos	206	2 bunches green onions
Mushrooms Barbacoa (×2)	196	2 cups fresh herbs (basil, cilantro, mint,
Peanut Slaw	114	or tarragon)
Barbacoa Mushroom Burritos	123	1½ cups alfalfa sprouts
Muesli	33	12 cups mixed greens

MONDAY

BREAKFAST
Muesli with nondairy milk
and fresh fruit

LUNCH
alfalfa sprouts and mixed
greens wrap with White
Bean–Miso Spread

DINNER
Pasta with Vegetables and
White Bean–Miso Spread
Fresh Spinach Salad

TUESDAY

BREAKFAST
Muesli with nondairy milk
and fresh fruit

LUNCH
Asian Noodle Soup
Fresh Spinach Salad

DINNER
Mushroom Tacos
Fresh Spinach Salad

WEDNESDAY

BREAKFAST
Muesli with nondairy milk
and fresh fruit

LUNCH
alfalfa sprouts and mixed
greens wrap with White
Bean–Miso Spread

DINNER
Barbacoa Mushroom Burritos
mixed greens salad with
All-Purpose Vinaigrette

THURSDAY

BREAKFAST
Muesli with nondairy milk
and fresh fruit

LUNCH
Beans and Grain Salad served
on a bed of mixed greens

DINNER
Asian Noodle Soup
mixed greens salad with
All-Purpose Vinaigrette

FRIDAY

BREAKFAST
Muesli with nondairy milk
and fresh fruit

LUNCH
Pasta with Vegetables and
White Bean–Miso Spread

DINNER
Portobello Mushroom
Burgers
mixed greens salad with
All-Purpose Vinaigrette

MENU PLAN III

Here's a good menu plan for stir-fry lovers. Stir-fry is one of my favorite meals, especially because it comes together so quickly once you have everything in place. You can vary the vegetables throughout the week and use either cooked rice or quinoa to serve with it. I also use leftover stir-fry to make a burrito that I can take for lunch. And I make extra Green Sauce to add to my burrito—delicious!!

Most days I make a smoothie for breakfast—it only takes five minutes. I vary the fruits each day and always keep a good supply of frozen fruit on hand. Muffins are an occasional treat and good to have on hand when making a smoothie is out of the question.

For this menu, you will need the recipes listed below, as well as the items in the additional ingredients list. See the pantry list on p. 21 for items you should always have on hand.

MAKE IT EASY:

- Keep Date and Soy Stir-Fry Sauce on hand.
- Make a double batch of the Orange-Miso Salad Dressing and pair it with the Apple, Fig, and Arugula Salad.
- If time is an issue, make quinoa in place of brown rice to use in your stir-fries and Falafel Bowl. It takes only 15 minutes to cook instead of the 45 minutes that brown rice takes.
- You can also buy minced garlic in a jar—1 teaspoon equals 1 clove.

MENU	ADDITIONAL INGREDIENTS
Blueberry Cornmeal Muffins 40	1 bunch bananas
Broccoli, Red Pepper, and Brown Rice	2 large apples, for muffins
Stir-Fry 183	1 large head green leaf lettuce or red leaf
Date and Soy Stir-Fry Sauce 61	lettuce, for sandwiches
Falafel Bowl 202	2 cups alfalfa sprouts
Green Sauce (×2) 52	2 red bell peppers
Falafel (×2) 82	2 cups mung bean sprouts
Falafel Tacos 205	8 cups fresh arugula
Apple, Fig, and Arugula Salad 89	2 large Fuji apples
All-Purpose Vinaigrette (×2) 44	2 bunches fresh kale
Fancy-Pants Chickpea Salad 108	2 bunches fresh cilantro
Basic Mayonnaise 53	6 cups mixed greens
Kale Salad with Orange-Miso	1 large tomato
Dressing 92	½ pound fresh asparagus
Orange-Miso Salad Dressing 48	1 8-ounce package sliced mushrooms
Almond Noodles 133	1 clove garlic
	1 small bunch fresh parsley
	6 dried figs
	1 large orange
	whole wheat lavash

MONDAY

BREAKFAST

Blueberry Cornmeal Muffins

LUNCH

Fancy-Pants Chickpea Salad sandwich on whole wheat buns with lettuce and sprouts

Kale Salad with Orange-Miso Dressing

DINNER

Broccoli, Red Pepper, and Brown Rice Stir-Fry

TUESDAY

BREAKFAST
Blueberry Cornmeal Muffins

LUNCH
Falafel Bowl
Kale Salad with Orange-Miso
   Dressing

DINNER
Broccoli, Red Pepper, and
   Brown Rice Stir-Fry
Apple, Fig, and Arugula Salad

WEDNESDAY

BREAKFAST
Smoothie

LUNCH
leftover stir-fry wrap
Apple, Fig, and Arugula Salad

DINNER
Broccoli, Red Pepper, and
   Brown Rice Stir-Fry
mixed greens salad with
   Orange-Miso Salad
   Dressing

THURSDAY

BREAKFAST
Smoothie

LUNCH
leftover stir-fry wrap

DINNER
Almond Noodles on mixed
   greens

FRIDAY

BREAKFAST
Smoothie

LUNCH
Almond Noodles on mixed
   greens

DINNER
Falafel Tacos

PANTRY LIST

ARROWROOT POWDER

BAKING POWDER

BAKING SODA

BEANS AND LEGUMES (CANNED AND DRIED)

adzuki beans, black beans, black-eyed peas, cannellini beans, garbanzo beans (chickpeas), navy beans, red kidney beans, red lentils, refried beans

BOTTLED LEMON JUICE

BUNS (WHOLE GRAIN)

burger buns, hoagie/submarine buns, sandwich buns

CANNED FRUITS AND VEGETABLES

applesauce, artichoke hearts, diced tomatoes, mandarin oranges, roasted red peppers, sweet potato puree, sun-dried tomatoes, tomato paste, tomato sauce

CONDIMENTS

brown rice syrup, capers, chipotle peppers in adobo sauce, dijon mustard, liquid aminos, maple syrup, marinara sauce, miso paste, olives in brine, pickle relish, sliced pickles, red hot sauce, salsa, soy sauce or tamari, silken tofu, nutritional yeast

FRUITS (DRIED)

apples, apricots, coconut (shredded), Medjool dates, raisins

FRUITS (FRESH AND/OR FROZEN)

apples, bananas, blueberries, figs, lemons, limes, mangoes, oranges, peaches, pears, pineapples, strawberries, tomatoes, watermelons

GRAINS

barley, brown rice, bulgur, cornmeal, quick-cooking oats, quinoa, rolled oats, rye

HERBS AND SPICES

ground allspice, ground black pepper, ground caraway, ancho chili powder, fresh and dried basil, dried bay leaf, cayenne pepper, fresh chives, cilantro, ground cinnamon, ground cloves, unsweetened cocoa, ground coriander, ground cumin, curry powder, fresh and dried dill, ground fennel seeds, granulated garlic, fresh and ground ginger, green onions, fresh and dried mint, mustard powder, ground nutmeg, granulated onion, dried oregano, sweet paprika, fresh parsley, crushed red pepper flakes, dried rosemary, saffron, dried sage, sea salt, star anise, dried tarragon, dried thyme, ground turmeric, vanilla extract

LIGHT COCONUT MILK

NUTS AND SEEDS

almonds, cashews, pecans, pine nuts, sunflower seeds, sesame seeds, walnuts

NUT BUTTERS

almond, cashew, peanut, tahini

PASTA (WHOLE GRAIN)

fettuccine, fusilli, linguine, macaroni, penne, rotini, spaghetti

PASTRY FLOUR (WHOLE WHEAT)

TORTILLAS

corn tortillas, whole wheat flour tortillas

THAI RED CURRY PASTE

UNSWEETENED NONDAIRY MILK

almond milk, rice milk, soy milk

VEGETABLES (FRESH AND/OR FROZEN)

arugula, avocados, bell peppers, bok choy, broccoli, carrots, cauliflower, celery, chard, corn, edamame, eggplants, garlic, green peas, jalapeño peppers, kale, leeks, lettuce, mushrooms, onions, poblano peppers, potatoes, serrano peppers, slaw mix, spinach, sweet potatoes, mixed vegetables, shallots, sprouts, zucchini

VEGETABLE STOCK

VINEGARS

apple cider vinegar, balsamic vinegar, red wine vinegar, rice wine vinegar, white wine vinegar

RECIPES

BREAKFAST DISHES

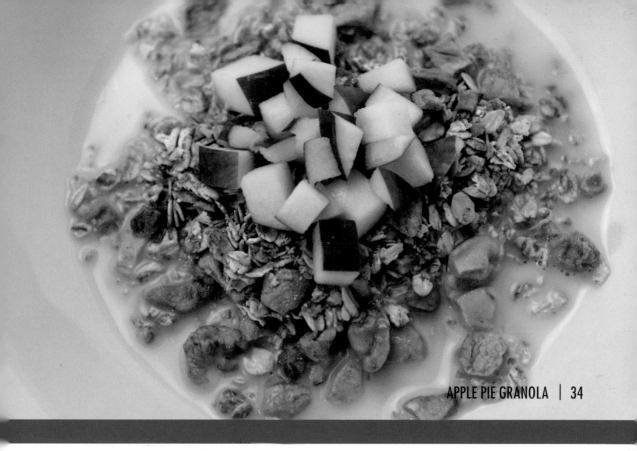

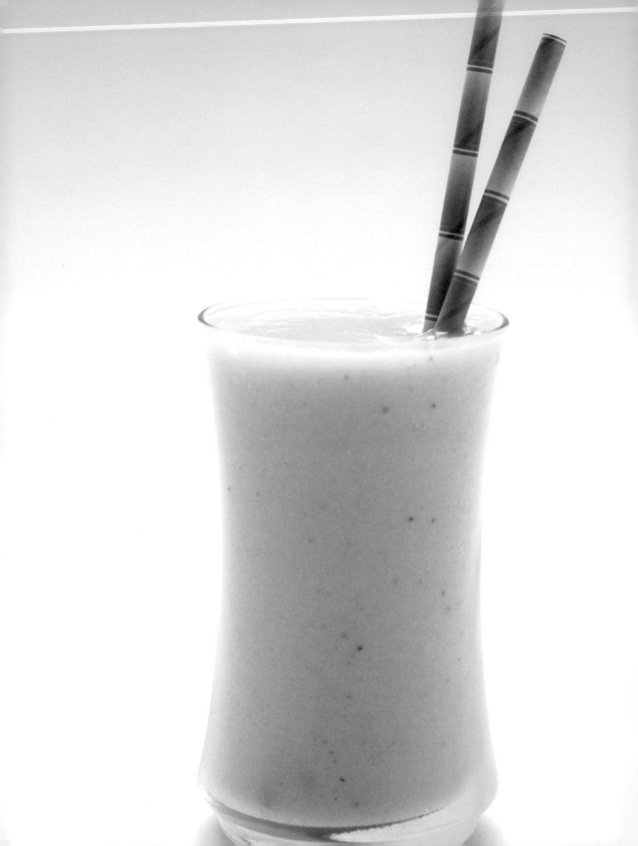

BANANA-PINEAPPLE SMOOTHIE

MAKES 1 SERVING

My first meal of the day is usually a smoothie and sometimes my midday meal might be another smoothie if I am in a hurry. I vary the flavors by changing the fruits. This recipe and the few that follow are some of my favorite smoothie recipes.

½ cup unsweetened nondairy milk, more as needed
1 large ripe banana, sliced
1½ cups frozen pineapple chunks
½ cup pitted Medjool dates or Two-Minute Date Puree (p. 62)
2 teaspoons lemon juice (optional)

1. Combine everything in a blender and process until smooth and creamy. Add more milk as necessary to achieve a pourable consistency.

MAKE IT EASY

I keep pineapple chunks and other fruits in the freezer so I can have this quick breakfast treat ready in a flash. If using fresh pineapple, blend 1 cup of pineapple chunks with 3 ice cubes.

STRAWBERRY CREAM SMOOTHIE

MAKES 1 SERVING

The strawberries and vanilla extract in this recipe make the smoothie taste like strawberry ice cream. You could also try almond extract for a little variety.

1 cup unsweetened nondairy milk, plus more as needed
1½ cups frozen strawberries
2–3 pitted Medjool dates, or to taste
½ teaspoon vanilla extract

1. Combine everything in a blender and process until smooth and creamy. Add more milk as necessary to achieve a pourable consistency.

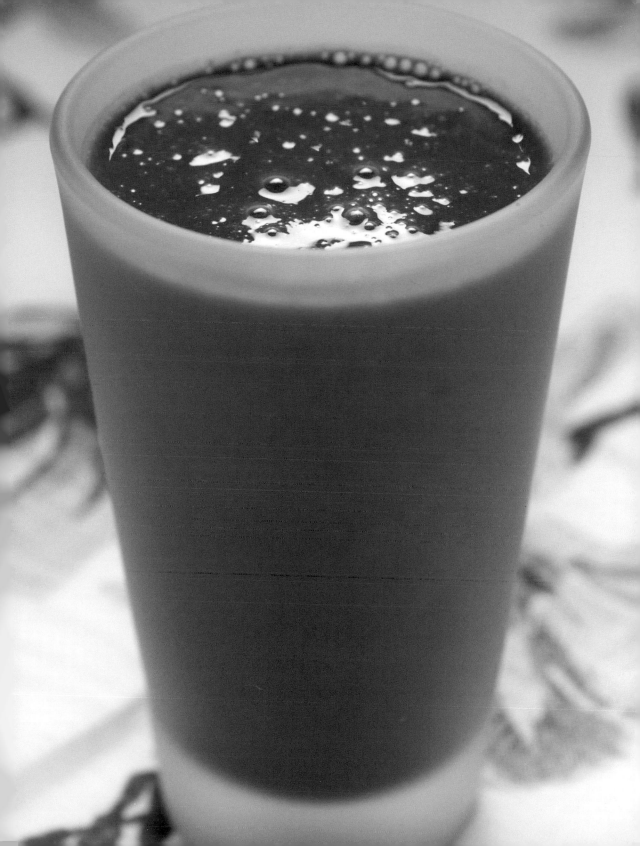

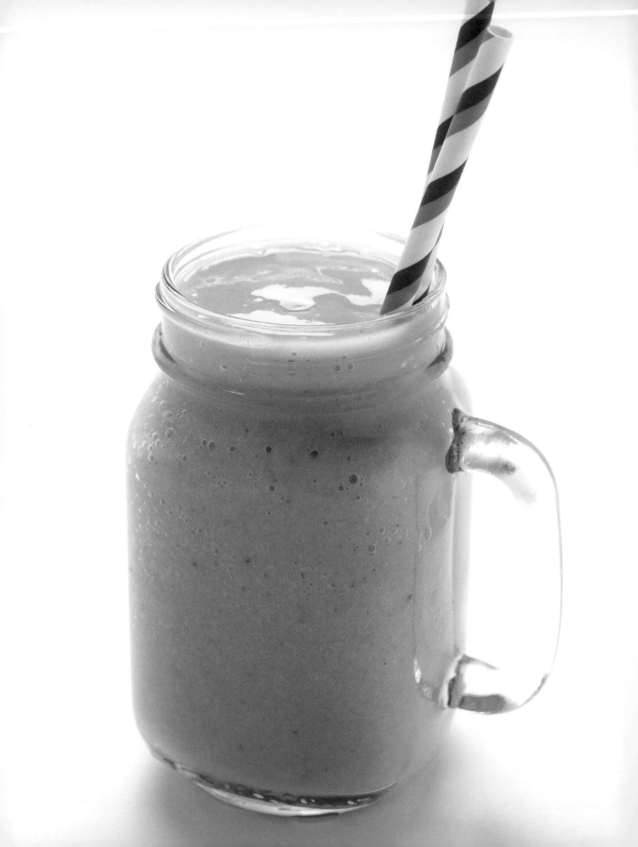

PEACH-MANGO SMOOTHIE

MAKES 1 SERVING

You'll never find peaches growing next to mangos where I come from, but they taste great together in a smoothie.

¾ cup frozen peach slices
¾ cup frozen mango chunks
1 cup unsweetened nondairy milk, plus more as needed
2–3 pitted Medjool dates, or to taste
½ teaspoon lemon juice

1. Combine everything in a blender and process until smooth and creamy. Add more milk as necessary to achieve a pourable consistency.

BANANA BREAD SMOOTHIE

MAKES 1 SERVING

The cinnamon, nutmeg, and vanilla extract really give this smoothie that banana bread flavor, so don't leave them out. Smoothies are like an instant breakfast. Keep ingredients on hand, have breakfast ready in less than five minutes, and never have an excuse to skip breakfast.

2 ripe bananas
1 cup unsweetened nondairy milk, plus more as needed
1 cup ice
2 tablespoons maple syrup or ¼ cup pitted Medjool dates
pinch ground cinnamon
pinch ground nutmeg
¼ teaspoon vanilla extract

1. Combine everything in a blender and process until smooth and creamy. Add more milk as necessary to achieve a pourable consistency.

MUESLI

Muesli is a breakfast cereal made from rolled oats, fresh and dried fruit, nuts and seeds, and sometimes other grains. It is easy to prepare and nice to have on hand since it keeps well in an airtight container. Try adding chopped fresh fruit and unsweetened nondairy milk.

3 cups rolled oats or other rolled grain like rye or barley
1 cup chopped dried fruit (raisins, apricots, figs, dates, apples, etc.)
½ cup chopped nuts or seeds (walnuts, pecans, cashews, almonds,
   sunflower seeds, sesame seeds, etc.)

1. Preheat the oven to 350°F.
2. Place the oats or grains on a baking sheet and toast them for 13–15 minutes, until they are lightly browned.
3. Remove the oats or grains from the oven and let them cool to room temperature.
4. Combine them with the remaining ingredients before serving, and store leftovers in an airtight container for up to 7 days.

APPLE PIE GRANOLA

MAKES 12 (¾-CUP) SERVINGS

I love making this granola in the summer when I don't want to turn the oven on. While not as crunchy as traditional baked granolas, it is just as flavorful. I eat it with a little nondairy milk and occasionally a chopped fresh apple or pear.

1 cup **Two-Minute Date Puree (p. 62)**
1 tablespoon ground cinnamon
1 teaspoon ground nutmeg
1 teaspoon sea salt
8 cups rolled oats
2 cups chopped dried apples, or to taste

1. Add the Two-Minute Date Puree, cinnamon, nutmeg, and sea salt to a large pot and mix well.
2. Bring the mixture to a boil over medium heat and add the rolled oats.
3. Cook for 5 minutes, stirring frequently until the Two-Minute Date Puree is absorbed and the oats start to brown.
4. Remove the pot from the stove and let it cool to room temperature.
5. Add the chopped dried apples, stir to mix, and store in an airtight container for up to 7 days.

> ## TIPS
>
> - For a crispier granola, you can bake it in the oven instead of cooking it on the stovetop. You will need to bake it at 325°F on a nonstick baking sheet for 35–40 minutes.
> - To serve, add ¾ cup of the granola to a bowl. Top with chopped fresh apple and unsweetened nondairy milk.

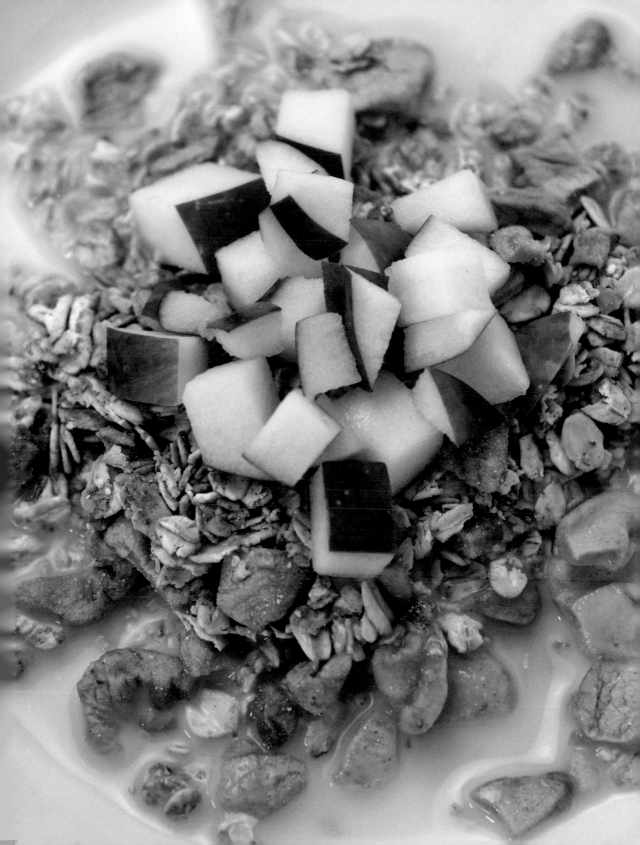

EASY CREAMY POLENTA

MAKES ABOUT 4 CUPS

Polenta, or cooked cornmeal, is an easy, versatile cereal, good for breakfast or any other meal. You can use this in any recipes calling for polenta in this book.

4 cups water
1 teaspoon salt
1 cup polenta or yellow cornmeal

1. Bring the water to a boil in a 2-quart pot over high heat.

2. Add the salt and whisk, slowly adding the polenta to the pot in a steady stream.

3. Reduce the heat to medium and continue whisking until the polenta thickens.

4. Cover the pan with a tight-fitting lid and let the polenta cook for 30 minutes, stirring every 10 minutes.

5. Serve the polenta as is or pour it into a loaf pan or baking dish and refrigerate until it sets. Once it sets, you can bake it on a parchment-lined baking sheet at 350°F for 15–20 minutes.

> ### TIP
>
> For a fun treat, make extra apple filling for Stovetop Fruit Crisp (p. 218) and serve it over the cooked polenta. You can also cook the polenta with chopped dried fruit and 1 teaspoon vanilla extract—delicious for breakfast or dessert.

OATMEAL-RAISIN BREAKFAST BARS

MAKES 12 BARS

I call these bars "breakfast on the go." When I am traveling, I take them in the car with me so I can have a quick, healthy breakfast or midday snack.

1¼ cups whole wheat pastry flour
1½ cups quick cooking oats
2 teaspoons baking powder
1 teaspoon ground cinnamon
½ teaspoon sea salt
1 cup unsweetened applesauce

1 cup unsweetened nondairy milk
½ cup natural peanut butter
¼ cup maple syrup
1 teaspoon vanilla extract
½ cup raisins

1. Preheat the oven to 350°F. Combine the flour, oats, baking powder, cinnamon, and sea salt in a mixing bowl.

2. In another bowl, combine the applesauce, nondairy milk, peanut butter, maple syrup, and vanilla and whisk well. Add it to the flour mixture with the raisins and gently fold to combine.

3. Press the batter into a parchment-lined or nonstick 9 × 13 baking dish and bake for 22–25 minutes, until a toothpick inserted in the center of the pan comes out clean.

4. Let the bars cool for 20 minutes before cutting into squares and serving. Store leftovers in an airtight container for 5 days.

MAKE IT EASY

- You can use Two-Minute Date Puree (p. 62) in place of the maple syrup—just increase the applesauce by ¼ cup.
- Use whatever nut butter you like in place of the peanut butter.
- If you want to make these bars lower in fat, leave out the peanut butter and use an equal amount of unsweetened applesauce in its place.
- Try different dried fruits in place of the raisins for a change.

SWEET POTATO PIE MUFFINS

MAKES 10 LARGE OR 14–16 SMALL MUFFINS

These muffins are based on my recipe for sweet potato pie. The orange zest, cinnamon, and allspice give the otherwise plain sweet potato a bright kick.

3 cups whole wheat pastry flour
4 teaspoons baking powder
1½ teaspoons ground cinnamon
½ teaspoon ground allspice
½ teaspoon sea salt
¾ cup sweet potato puree
2 cups unsweetened nondairy milk
2 teaspoons apple cider vinegar
¼ cup maple syrup or Two-Minute Date Puree (p. 62)
zest of 1 orange

1. Preheat the oven to 350°F.
2. Line the cups of a muffin pan with paper liners.
3. Combine the flour, baking powder, cinnamon, allspice, and sea salt in a mixing bowl and mix well.
4. In a separate bowl, combine the sweet potato puree, nondairy milk, apple cider vinegar, maple syrup or Two-Minute Date Puree, and orange zest. Mix well.
5. Add the sweet potato mixture to the flour mixture and gently fold together.
6. Divide the batter between the muffin tins and bake for 20–25 minutes, until a toothpick inserted in the center of the muffins comes out clean.

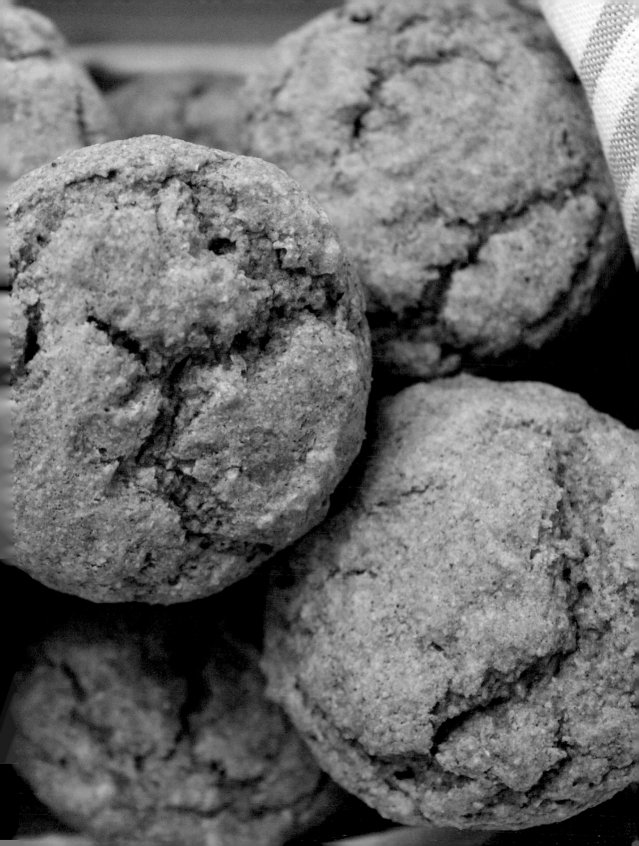

FRESH APPLE MUFFINS

MAKES 10 LARGE OR 14–16 SMALL MUFFINS

The key to oil-free baking is the lightness of touch. Do not overmix the ingredients and do measure ingredients exactly to get moist and light baked goods.

3 cups whole wheat pastry flour
1½ teaspoons baking powder
1½ teaspoons baking soda
1 teaspoon ground cinnamon
½ teaspoon ground nutmeg

3 cups grated apples
1 cup unsweetened applesauce
¾ cup unsweetened nondairy milk
¼ cup maple syrup or Two-Minute
    Date Puree (p. 62)

1. Preheat the oven to 350°F.
2. Line the cups of a muffin pan with paper liners.
3. Combine the flour, baking powder, baking soda, cinnamon, and nutmeg in a bowl and whisk to mix well.
4. Add the remaining ingredients to the bowl and, using a spoon or spatula, fold the wet ingredients into the dry ingredients.
5. Fill each muffin cup ⅔ full.
6. Bake the muffins for 20 minutes, until a toothpick inserted in the center of the muffin comes out clean.

VARIATION — BLUEBERRY CORNMEAL MUFFINS

Replace 1 cup of the whole wheat pastry flour with cornmeal, add 1 cup of fresh blueberries, and reduce the grated apples to 2 cups.

> **TIP**
>
> I like Granny Smith apples for the tart flavor they add to this muffin.

STOVETOP RICE PUDDING

MAKES 4 SERVINGS

I am one of those people who will eat plain brown rice with salt and pepper, but this dish makes me feel like I won a prize that I didn't have to do much to earn. If you make a big pot of brown rice at the beginning of the week, you can use leftovers to make this recipe for breakfast—or dessert.

4½ cups cooked brown rice
1 cup golden raisins or other dried fruit
   (chopped if large, like apricots)
⅓ cup Two-Minute Date Puree (p. 62) or maple
   syrup

1½ cups unsweetened nondairy milk
½ cup toasted chopped almonds (optional)
2 teaspoons ground cinnamon
1 teaspoon vanilla or almond extract
sea salt to taste

1. Combine everything in a medium saucepan and simmer over medium heat for 10 minutes or until thickened.

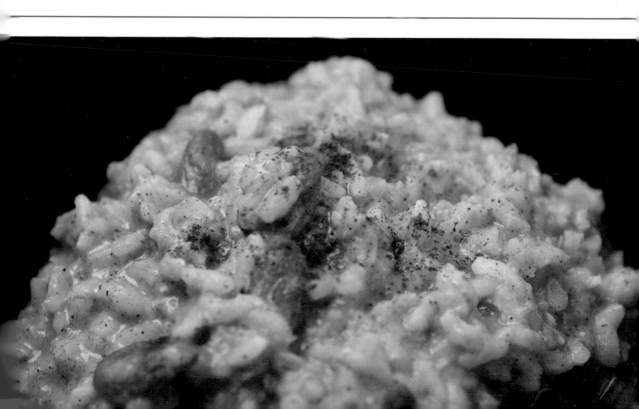

SAUCES,
SALAD DRESSINGS
& SEASONINGS

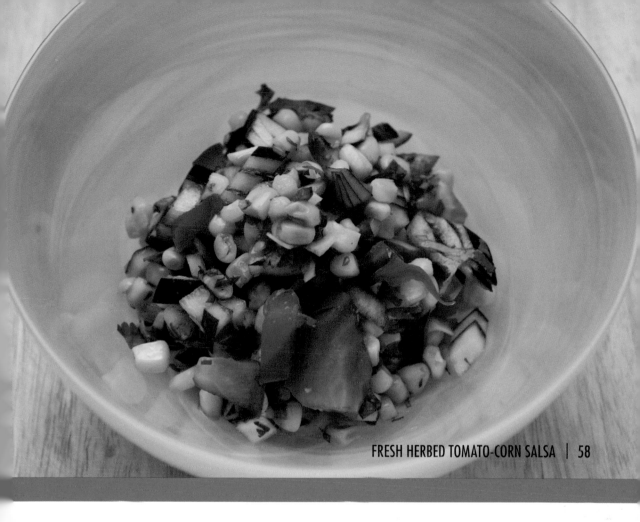

ALL-PURPOSE VINAIGRETTE

MAKES ¾ CUP

Make this easy oil-free dressing in large batches to have on hand for a number of uses. It is a perfect salad dressing for mixed greens or romaine lettuce and can be used as a dressing for the Beans and Grain Salad (p. 103) or Black-Eyed Pea Salad (p. 110).

½ cup balsamic vinegar
¼ cup Dijon mustard
¼ cup minced shallot
black pepper to taste

1. Combine all ingredients in a small bowl and mix well. Store refrigerated in an airtight container for up to 7 days.

ASIAN SALAD DRESSING

MAKES 1¼ CUPS

Soy, ginger, garlic, and rice vinegar are classic ingredients in a wide variety of Asian foods. This dressing is full of flavor and makes a great marinade for vegetables.

½ cup rice vinegar

½ cup brown rice syrup

¼ cup low-sodium soy sauce or tamari

1 teaspoon ground ginger

1 teaspoon garlic powder

1. Combine everything in a small bowl and whisk to mix well. Store refrigerated in an airtight container for up to 10 days.

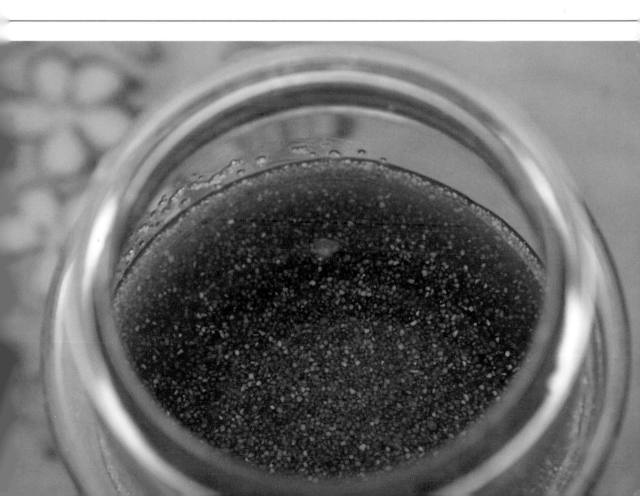

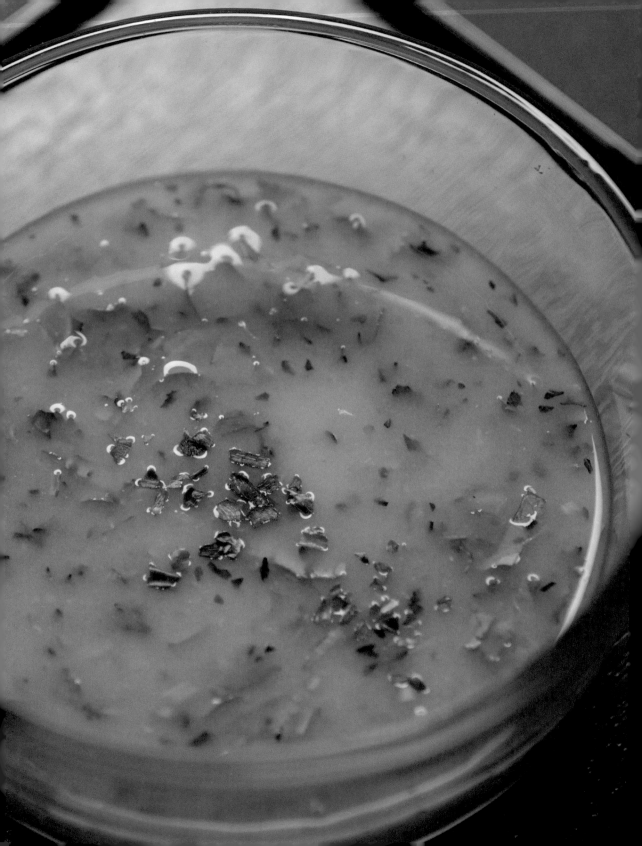

HERBED ORANGE VINAIGRETTE

MAKES 1 CUP

Now and then I need a change from the usual vinaigrettes for my salads, and this is one of my favorites. It is light, easy, and versatile. I often make this salad dressing with my Two-Minute Date Puree in place of rice syrup to make a dressing free of processed sugar, but it makes a visually less appealing salad dressing.

⅓ cup orange juice
⅓ cup brown rice syrup or Two-Minute Date Puree (p. 62)
⅓ cup white wine vinegar
2 teaspoons Dijon mustard
¼ cup chopped fresh cilantro
1½ teaspoons dried mint
½ teaspoon crushed red pepper flakes

1. Combine all ingredients in a bowl and whisk to mix well. Store refrigerated in an airtight container for up to 10 days.

ORANGE-MISO SALAD DRESSING

MAKES 1 CUP

I love this citrusy variation of a classic Asian dressing. The added kick from the ginger and cayenne pepper will liven up any salad.

½ cup bottled orange juice (not from concentrate)
1 tablespoon grated fresh ginger
¼ cup mellow white miso paste (also known as sweet miso)
¼ cup rice wine vinegar
½ teaspoon cayenne pepper (optional)

1. Combine everything in a blender and process until smooth and creamy. Store refrigerated in an airtight container for up to 7 days.

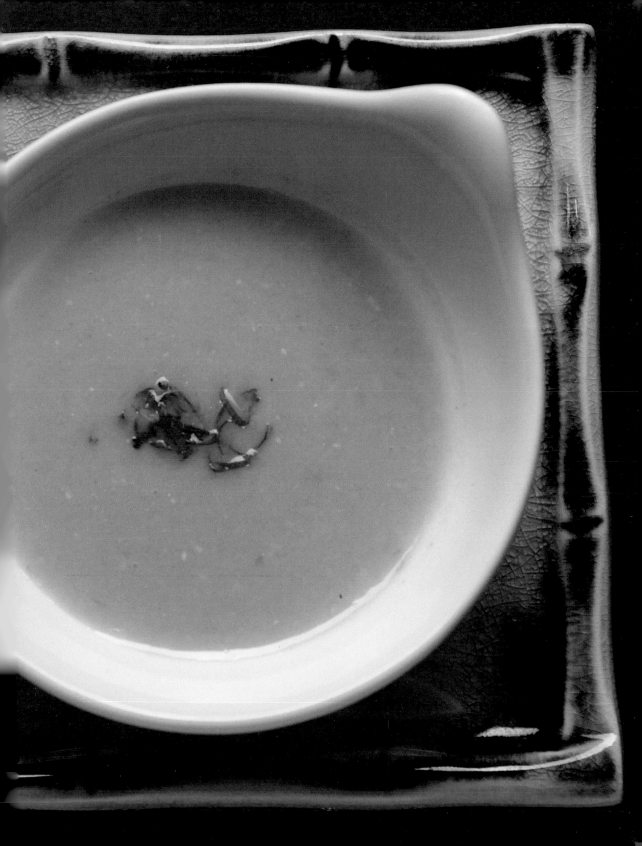

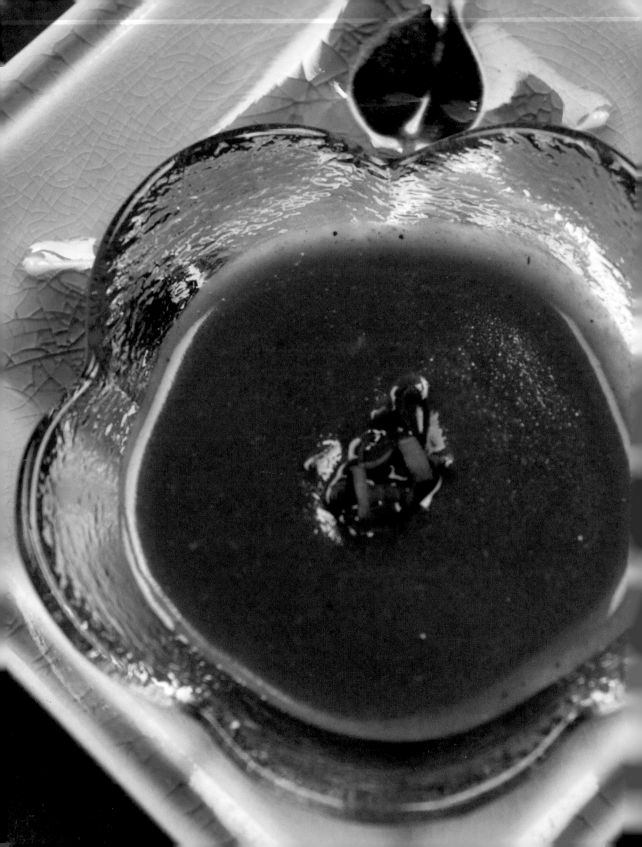

ALMOST INSTANT PEANUT SAUCE

MAKES ABOUT 1 CUP

The ginger and cayenne give this sauce a flavorful kick, and it takes only 5 minutes to make. Serve it with Warm Kale Salad with Peanut Dressing (p. 96), Chilled Peanut Noodles (p. 130), or Quinoa–Black Bean Buddha Bowl (p. 201).

½ cup smooth peanut butter
¼ cup low-sodium soy sauce or tamari
2 tablespoons rice vinegar
¼ cup brown rice syrup
¾ teaspoon ground ginger
¼ teaspoon cayenne pepper (optional)

1. Combine all ingredients in a bowl and whisk well to combine. Store refrigerated in an airtight container for up to 7 days.

GREEN SAUCE

MAKES 1¾ CUPS

I used to make a version of this sauce with sesame oil and tahini. It was delicious, but heavy. Now I love it without the sesame oil, and you could make this flavor-packed version even lower in fat by leaving out the tahini (see Tip). You will still have a really good sauce to use on pasta, steamed vegetables, or many other dishes you'll find in this book.

1 12-ounce package Mori-Nu Silken Lite Firm Tofu
¾ cup chopped fresh cilantro
¼ cup tahini (not raw)
2 tablespoons lemon juice
4 cloves garlic
2 teaspoons sea salt
¼ teaspoon cayenne pepper

1. Combine all ingredients in a blender and puree until smooth and creamy.
2. Store refrigerated in an airtight container for up to 7 days.

> ### TIP
>
> If you leave out the tahini, increase the cilantro to 1 cup.

BASIC MAYONNAISE

MAKES 1½ CUPS

I prefer to make my mayonnaise with cauliflower puree instead of tofu, not only because I have a mild allergy to soy but because I like the taste better—and the cauliflower has no fat. But whether you use tofu or cauliflower, this recipe will keep refrigerated for seven days.

1 12-ounce package Mori-Nu Silken Lite Firm Tofu or
    1½ cups Cauliflower Puree (p. 64)
2 tablespoons red wine vinegar
½ teaspoon sea salt

1. Combine everything in a food processor or blender and puree until smooth and creamy.

MAKE IT EASY

I keep this recipe on hand as my starter mayonnaise, then I can add whatever I like to it depending upon what I am making—roasted red peppers, Dijon mustard, fresh or dried herbs, or garlic.

RED PEPPER MAYO

MAKES 2 CUPS

I love roasted red bell peppers. When you puree them and put them in a mayonnaise like this one, their flavor intensifies. I use this sauce to make Red Pepper Slaw (p. 113) or as a condiment for sandwiches.

1½ cups Cauliflower Puree (p. 64) or
   1 12-ounce package Mori-Nu Silken Lite Firm Tofu
2 roasted red bell peppers
2 tablespoons red wine vinegar
1 tablespoon chopped fresh dill
sea salt and black pepper to taste

1. Add the Cauliflower Puree or tofu to a blender with the remaining ingredients. Blend until smooth and creamy.

2. Store refrigerated in an airtight container for up to 5 days.

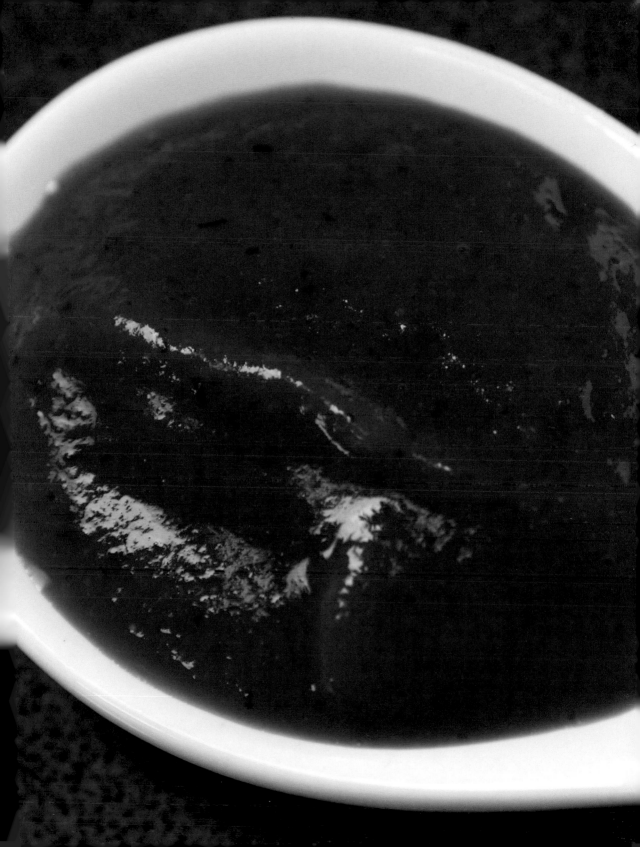

DEL'S FAVORITE PARMESAN

MAKES 1 CUP

There are many versions of vegan Parmesan cheese recipes and most of them are good—and pretty much the same. This is my favorite. The caraway and fennel seeds, just a touch of each, add a little brightness that reminds me of a good Parmesan.

¼ cup toasted sesame seeds
¼ cup toasted cashews
½ cup nutritional yeast
½ teaspoon sea salt
¼ teaspoon ground caraway seeds
¼ teaspoon ground fennel seeds

1. Combine all ingredients in a food processor and process until the mixture has the texture of grated Parmesan cheese. Do not over-process or you will have Parmesan butter.

2. Store refrigerated for up to 1 month.

JERK SPICE RUB

MAKES ¾ CUP

I love jerk seasonings. They are spicy, sweet, and pungent all at the same time. Making your own spice rub gives you some healthy advantages over buying commercial versions—you can determine how much heat you add to the rub and you can make it healthy by using the natural sweetness of dates instead of processed sugars. Use this delicious rub with Jerk-Style Beans (p. 188), baked or grilled portobello mushrooms, or cauliflower steaks.

½ cup water
4 Medjool dates, pitted
1 tablespoon granulated onion
1 tablespoon granulated garlic
1 tablespoon ground allspice
1 tablespoon dried thyme leaves
1 teaspoon sea salt
1 teaspoon cayenne pepper
½ teaspoon black pepper
½ teaspoon ground nutmeg

1. Combine all ingredients in a blender and puree until smooth and creamy.
2. Store refrigerated in an airtight container for up to 5 days.

FRESH HERBED TOMATO-CORN SALSA PICTURED ON PAGE 43

MAKES ABOUT 3½ CUPS

I make this recipe whenever tomatoes and corn are fresh at the farmers' market. It is great on Tostadas (p. 207), tossed in Penne with Fresh Herbed Tomato-Corn Salsa (p. 136), or as a side dish.

1 10-ounce package frozen corn or
   4 ears fresh corn, cut from the cob
1 large ripe tomato, diced
½ medium red onion, diced small
1 jalapeño pepper, seeded and diced
3 tablespoons balsamic vinegar
2 tablespoons chopped fresh basil
2 tablespoons chopped fresh cilantro
sea salt to taste

1. Combine everything in a large bowl and mix well. Let sit for 1 hour at room temperature or refrigerated to let the flavors marry.

> **TIP**
>
> You can also make this with just the basil or just the cilantro—but I like using both.

EASY DATE BARBECUE SAUCE

MAKES 3½ CUPS

Most commercial barbecue sauces are full of high fructose corn syrup or sugar. This recipe has neither and still delivers all of the flavors you want in your barbecue.

1 15-ounce can tomato puree
2 cups Two-Minute Date Puree (p. 62), more or less to taste
3 tablespoons prepared mustard
1 tablespoon apple cider or red wine vinegar
2 teaspoons paprika
1 teaspoon ground coriander
1 teaspoon cayenne pepper, more or less to taste

1. Combine everything in a small saucepan. Cook over medium-low heat, stirring often, for 10 minutes.
2. Store refrigerated in an airtight container for up to 10 days.

> **TIP**
>
> This sauce is less sweet than traditional barbecue sauces. You could add a few drops of stevia to make the difference.

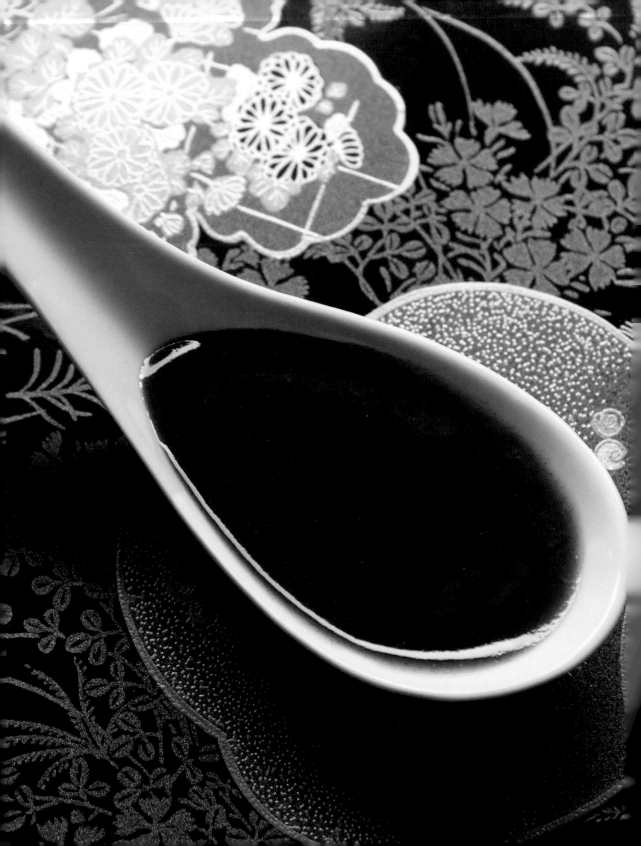

DATE AND SOY STIR-FRY SAUCE

MAKES 2 CUPS

I always have this sauce on hand. With this sauce, some cooked rice or pasta, and a package of frozen vegetables, I can have dinner ready in less than 15 minutes. Even if I have to make this easy sauce, I can have dinner in less than 30 minutes.

¼ cup low-sodium soy sauce or tamari, or to taste
1½ cups low-sodium vegetable stock
¼ cup pitted Medjool dates
1½ teaspoons ground ginger
1½ teaspoons granulated garlic
1 tablespoon arrowroot powder

1. Combine everything but the arrowroot powder in a saucepan and cook over medium heat for 5 minutes or until the dates are softened.

2. Add the cooked mixture to a blender and, with the motor running, add the arrowroot powder.

3. Store refrigerated in an airtight container for up to 7 days.

TWO-MINUTE DATE PUREE

MAKES 2½ CUPS

Two-Minute Date Puree is a great alternative to processed sugars, and this version doesn't require you to soak the dates. Medjool dates work best for this puree. They are sweeter, and if you can find fresh dates, they are creamier, but use what you can find. Even pitted dates sometimes have pits, so check them before you put them in the blender.

2 cups Medjool dates, pitted
2 cups water

1. Combine the dates and water in a blender and puree until smooth.
2. Store refrigerated for up to 7 days or in the freezer for up to 3 months.

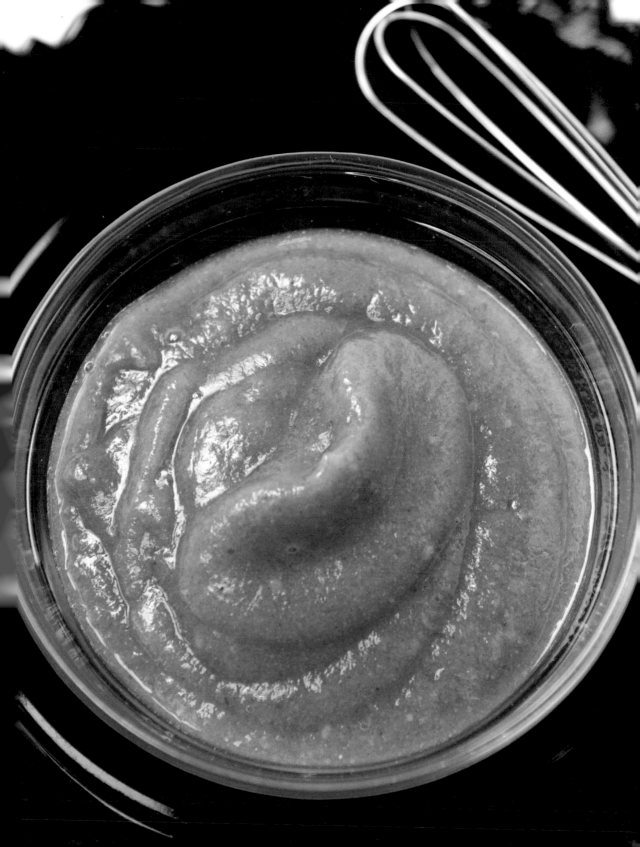

CAULIFLOWER PUREE

MAKES 2 CUPS ❄

I discovered this puree some years ago when I made a roasted cauliflower bisque for a holiday menu. The pureed cauliflower was so flavorful, I decided to use it as a cream sauce and have been using it ever since. I keep frozen cauliflower on hand, so this recipe only takes about 10 minutes. You can use silken tofu in place of the cauliflower for a similar sauce, especially if you are in a hurry, but give this puree a try. It is worth the effort.

2 cups fresh or frozen cauliflower florets
2 cups water

1. Combine the water and cauliflower in a small pan and cook over medium heat, covered, until the cauliflower is very tender, about 6 minutes for frozen or 10 minutes for fresh.

2. Drain the cauliflower, reserving any remaining cooking liquid.

3. Puree the cauliflower with enough of the reserved cooking liquid to make a creamy consistency.

4. Store refrigerated in an airtight container for up to 5 days.

SAFFRON CREAM

MAKES 3 CUPS

I love cream sauces—the rich flavor, the creamy mouthfeel, the versatility. This is one of my favorite cream sauces ever. I love saffron and pine nuts, and the two together make sauces with flavors right out of a Mediterranean bistro. Use this in Pasta with Saffron Cream (p. 147), or in unusual baked dishes like Baked Quinoa with Saffron Cream (p. 159) or Scalloped Potatoes with Saffron Cream (p. 156).

1 12-ounce package frozen cauliflower florets
2 cups vegetable stock
4 cloves garlic, minced
2 teaspoons granulated onion
2 teaspoons dried thyme
large pinch saffron
¼ cup toasted pine nuts
sea salt and black pepper to taste

1. Combine the cauliflower and the vegetable stock in a saucepan and cook for 8 minutes, until the cauliflower is tender.
2. Add the cauliflower and stock to a blender with the remaining ingredients and puree until smooth and creamy. Taste for sea salt and black pepper.

TIP

If you want a lower-fat sauce, the pine nuts are optional—but worth it for an occasional treat!

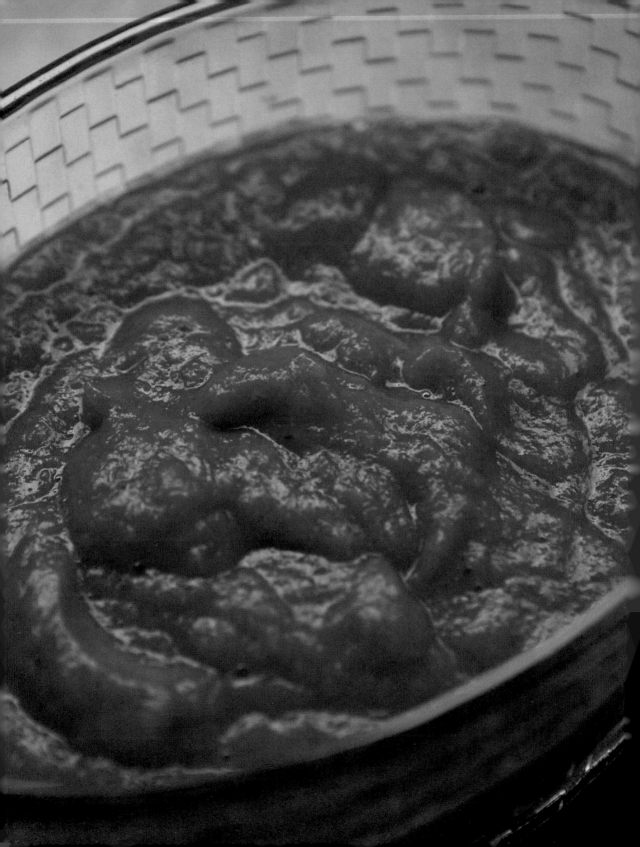

NO-QUESO SAUCE

MAKES ABOUT 3 CUPS

When I want a creamy sauce with a kick, I make this one. It can be used to make a great mac and cheese, No-Queso Mac and Cheese (p. 152); a fun version of scalloped potatoes, No-Queso Potato Bake (p. 155); or even as a sauce for burritos, Barbacoa Mushroom Burritos (p. 123).

2 cups frozen cauliflower florets
2 cups water
1 roasted red bell pepper
2 chipotle peppers in adobo sauce
1 teaspoon sea salt

1. Add the cauliflower to a medium saucepan with the water.
2. Bring to a boil over high heat and cook until the cauliflower is tender—6 minutes for the frozen; 10 minutes for the fresh.
3. Scoop the cauliflower into a blender, reserving the cooking liquid, and add the remaining ingredients.
4. Puree the mixture, adding just enough of the cooking water to make a creamy sauce.

MAKE IT EASY

You can make a quick, no-cook version of this sauce by replacing the cauliflower with light firm silken tofu and pureeing it with the rest of the ingredients. It makes a great dip for vegetables.

ALFREDO SAUCE

MAKES ABOUT 2½ CUPS

I used to make pasta Alfredo for a good friend of mine who proclaimed it "the best ever." Of course, it was full of dairy and fat. This sauce is just as rich as the original but dairy free and much lower in fat. It tastes great on Pasta Alfredo (p. 151), Pita Pizza Alfredo (p. 212), or a plain baked potato.

2 cups Cauliflower Puree (p. 64) or
   1 12-ounce package Mori-Nu Silken Lite Firm Tofu
1 cup Del's Favorite Parmesan (p. 56)
½ teaspoon ground nutmeg
sea salt and black pepper to taste

1. Add the Cauliflower Puree, Parmesan, and nutmeg to a blender and blend until smooth and creamy.
2. Add water as needed to make a creamy consistency. Season with sea salt and black pepper to taste.

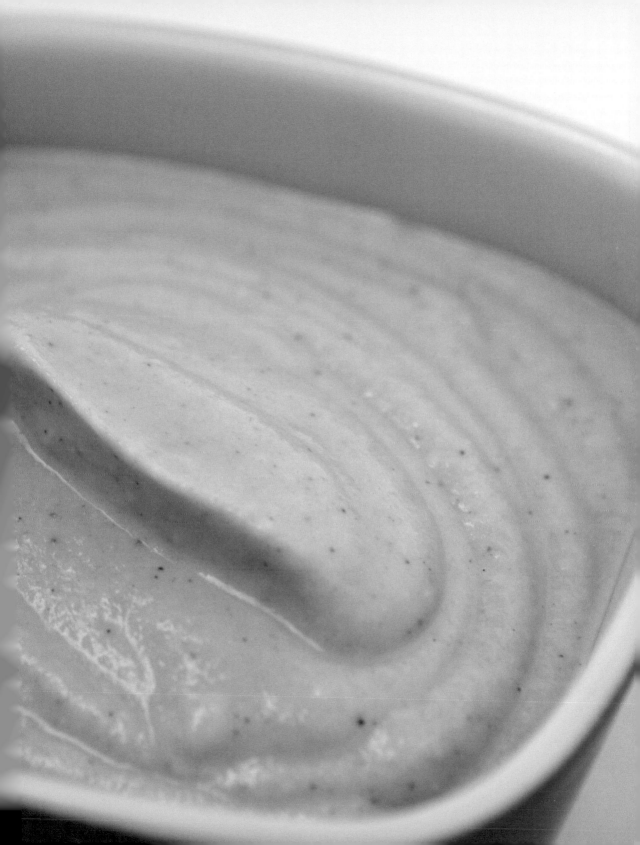

SNACKS & SPREADS

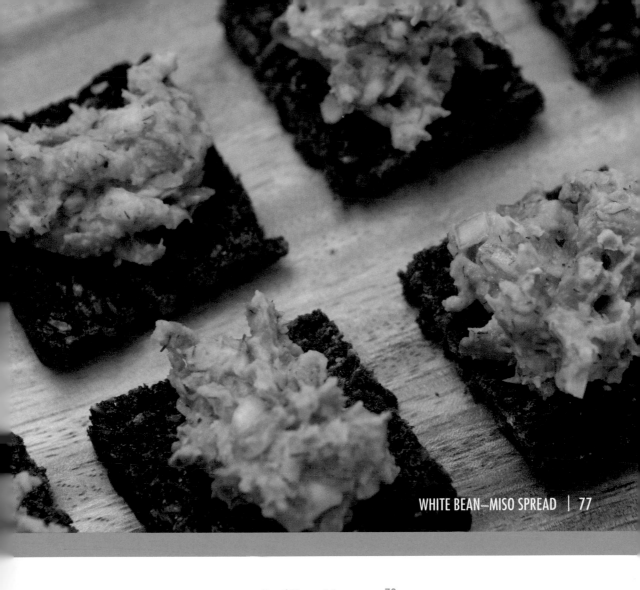

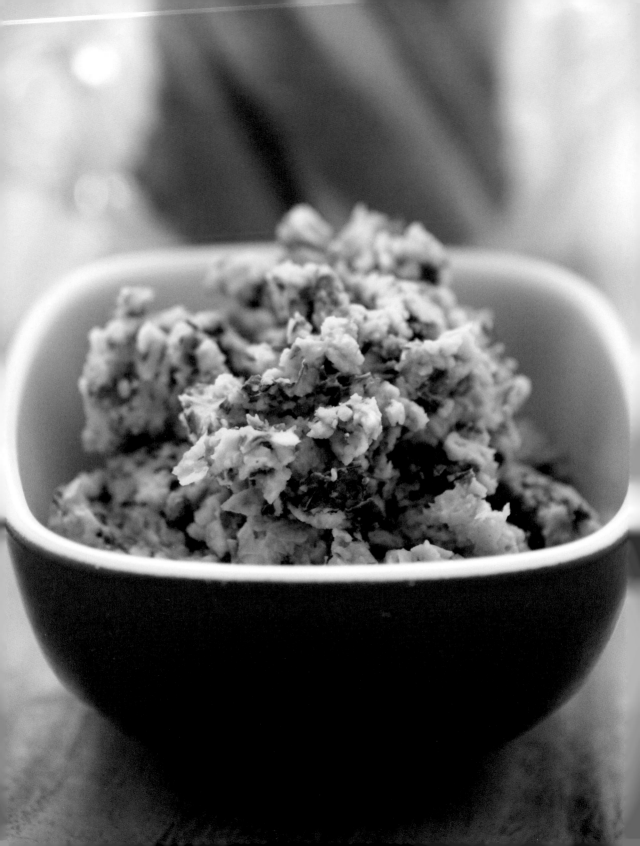

BASIL PESTO HUMMUS

MAKES 2 CUPS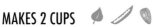

This recipe combines the best of two of my favorite recipes: pesto and hummus. It's almost like they belong together. I eat this as a snack with rice crackers or cucumber or celery slices, or on a sandwich with alfalfa sprouts and lettuce. The creamier you make this sauce, the more you will bring out the flavor of the basil and pine nuts, but a chunkier hummus is also good.

1 15-ounce can garbanzo beans (chickpeas), drained and rinsed
2 cups fresh basil leaves
¼ cup toasted pine nuts (optional)
juice of 1 lemon or 2 tablespoons lemon juice
2 cloves garlic, minced
1 teaspoon sea salt, more or less to taste
water as needed

1. Combine everything in a food processor and puree until smooth and creamy. Add a little water if needed to reach the desired consistency.

ROASTED RED PEPPER DIP

MAKES 4–6 SERVINGS

I love this creamy dip with fresh vegetables or as a sauce for veggie wraps. My favorite way to eat it, however, is to spread a thin layer on whole grain sandwich bread with maple-dijon Glazed Eggplant Cutlets (p. 195) and lettuce.

1 15-ounce can cannellini or navy beans, drained and rinsed
2 tablespoons almond butter
4 tablespoons mellow white miso paste
2 roasted red bell peppers
3 cloves garlic
2 tablespoons chopped fresh dill

1. Place all ingredients into the bowl of a food processor and blend until smooth and creamy.

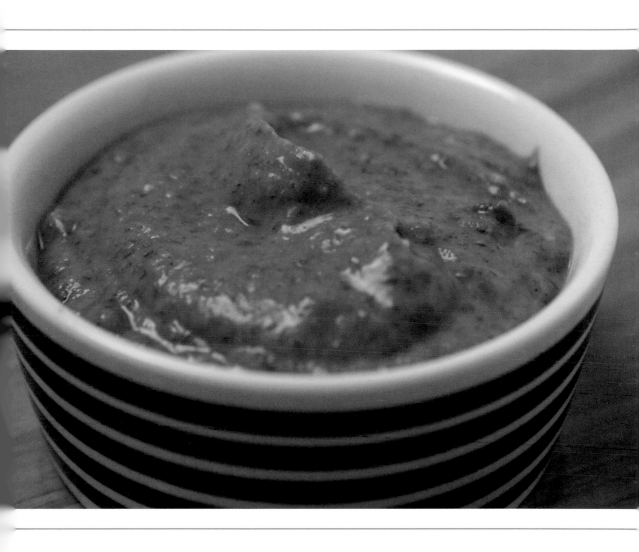

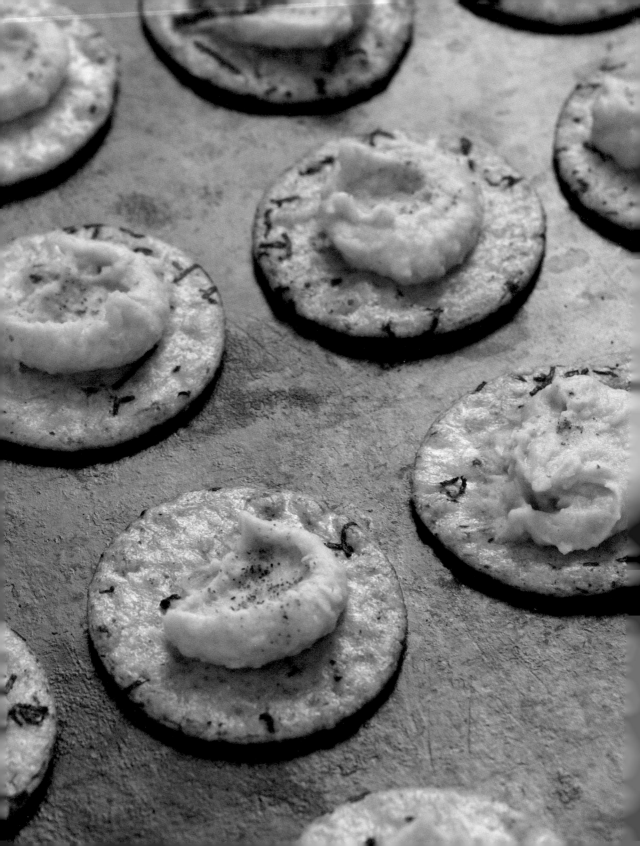

WHITE BEAN–MISO SPREAD

MAKES 4–6 SERVINGS

I used to make a lot of spreads with tofu, but after having a friend ask me to make her a spread with beans instead, I found that I liked it just as well. Now I often make my spreads with beans, and this is one of my favorites. I eat it in wraps with sprouts or fresh spinach, with celery sticks for a quick snack, and even as a sauce for dishes like Pasta with Vegetables and White Bean–Miso Spread (p. 144).

1 15-ounce can white beans (navy, great Northern,
    or cannellini), drained and rinsed
3 tablespoons mellow white miso paste
2 tablespoons almond butter (optional)
3 cloves garlic, minced
2 teaspoons granulated onion
½ teaspoon cayenne pepper (optional)

1. Add all ingredients to the bowl of a food processor and puree until smooth and creamy.

CARROT-ALMOND SPREAD

MAKES 4 SERVINGS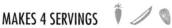

Toasted almonds add a nice crunch to this spread, and the grated carrots add a touch of sweetness. You might think that all beans taste the same, but you'd be mistaken. Try this with your favorite white bean, or try it with cooked adzuki beans or black-eyed peas for a change.

1 15-ounce can white beans (navy, great Northern,
   or cannellini), drained and rinsed
3 tablespoons mellow white miso paste
3 cloves garlic, minced
1 large carrot, grated (about 1½ cups)
1 small red onion, finely chopped (about ½ cup)
⅓ cup toasted chopped almonds
¼ cup chopped fresh dill

1. Add the beans, miso, and garlic to the bowl of a food processor and puree until smooth and creamy.

2. Add the bean mixture to a bowl with the remaining ingredients and mix well.

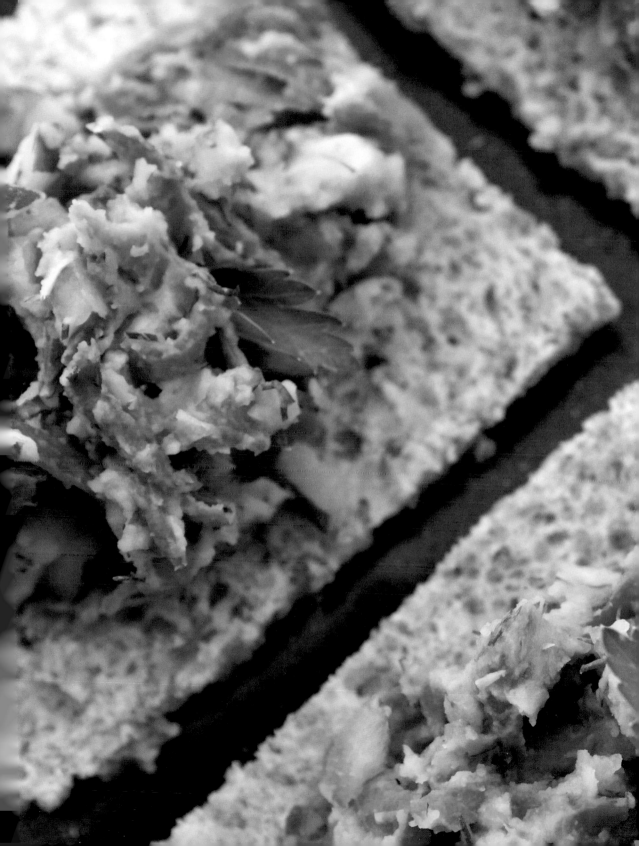

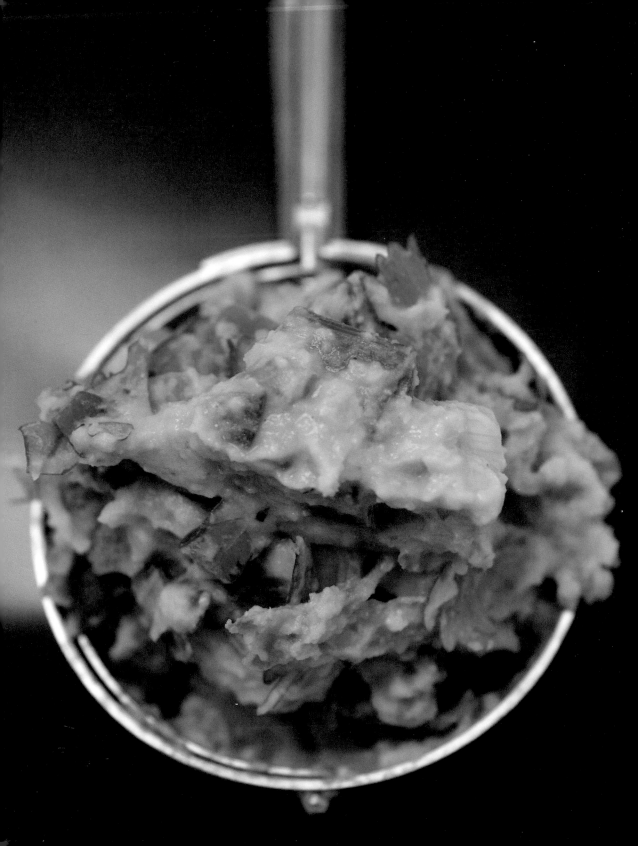

THAI BEAN SPREAD

MAKES 6 SERVINGS

I always crave this spread when it is cold outside. I eat it with crackers or on whole wheat bread with sprouts.

1 15-ounce can garbanzo beans (chickpeas), drained and rinsed
3 tablespoons almond butter (optional)
¼ cup lime juice
2 tablespoons low-sodium soy sauce or tamari, more or less to taste
1 medium carrot, grated
1 Thai red chili or 1 small jalapeño pepper, seeded and minced (optional)
¼ cup sliced green onion
¼ cup finely chopped fresh cilantro
2 cloves garlic, minced

1. Combine the garbanzo beans, almond butter, lime juice, and soy sauce in a food processor and process until smooth and creamy.
2. Spoon the mixture into a mixing bowl; add the remaining ingredients and mix well.

FALAFEL

MAKES 4 SERVINGS

I love falafel. I eat them as an appetizer, in a pita with Green Sauce (p. 52), or even on pizza. But I don't want all the added fat that would normally be in a deep-fried dish. So, I bake it instead and the results taste as good as the fried original.

2 15-ounce cans garbanzo beans (chickpeas), drained and rinsed
1 medium yellow onion, chopped
6 cloves garlic, chopped
4 tablespoons fresh parsley, chopped

1 tablespoon arrowroot powder
4 teaspoons ground coriander
2 teaspoons ground cumin
sea salt and black pepper to taste

1. Preheat the oven to 375°F.
2. Add everything to a food processor and process, leaving a little texture to the beans.
3. Using a small ice cream scoop or tablespoon, shape the mixture into balls. Place on a nonstick baking sheet and bake for 10 minutes.
4. Turn the falafel over and bake for another 8–10 minutes.

VARIATION — BREAKFAST FALAFEL PATTIES

Follow steps 1 and 2 in the recipe above, adding ½ teaspoon of ground fennel seeds and ½ teaspoon of crushed red pepper flakes. Using a small ice cream scoop or tablespoon, shape the mixture into balls. Place them on a nonstick baking sheet and press them to ½-inch thickness. Bake them as above.

MAKE IT EASY

If you happen to have baked sweet potatoes on hand, you can use them in place of the garbanzo beans. You'll need 1¾ cups of mashed sweet potatoes. The added sweetness of the earthy potatoes makes great falafel, and it's a nice way to sneak another serving of vegetables into your family's food.

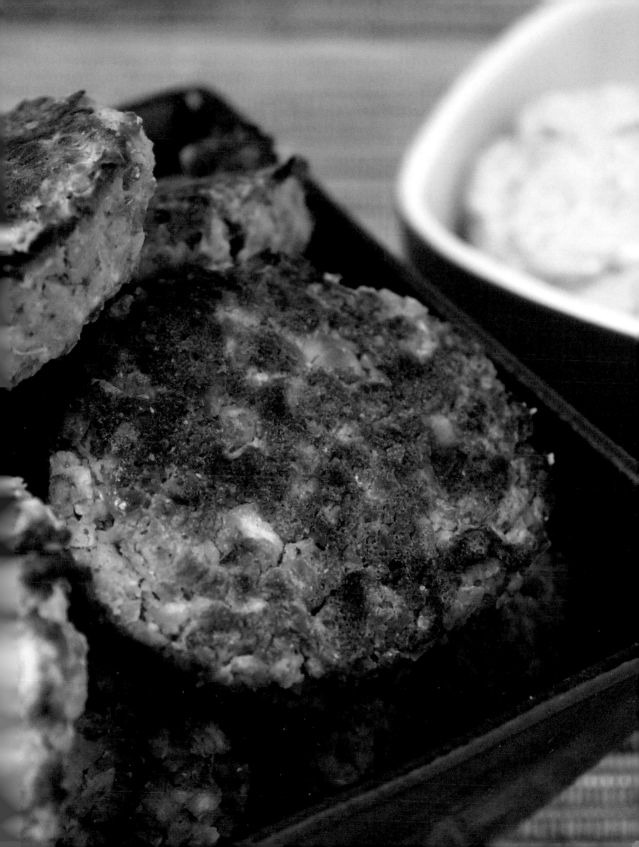

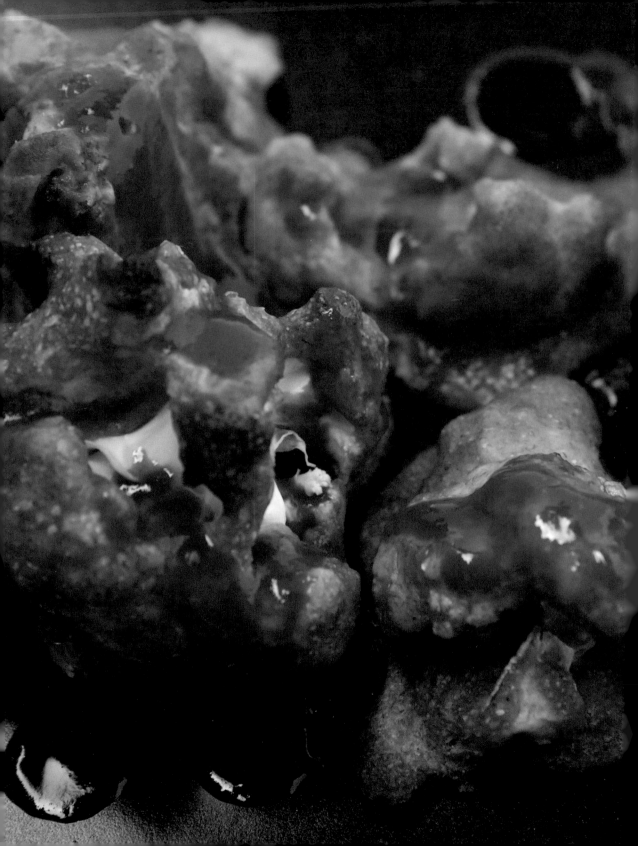

BUFFALO CAULIFLOWER BITES

MAKES 4–6 SERVINGS ✸

One of the unhealthy things I inherited from my grandmother was her deep fryer—and I used to use it a lot, mostly to make buffalo wings. Now I want a healthier snack but I still love that hot spicy sauce—I just want it without the added oil, and I really don't want the wings. Buffalo Cauliflower Bites do the trick! They are full of flavor and spice without all the bad stuff. One of my favorite sandwiches to make is a Buffalo Po' Boy (p. 119) on a whole grain hoagie bun (or sandwich bun) with Peanut Slaw (p. 114).

½ cup water
¼ cup almond butter
½ cup red hot sauce, plus extra for tossing with the cooked bites
¾ cup whole wheat pastry flour
¼ cup nutritional yeast
1½ tablespoons granulated garlic
1 large head cauliflower, cut into 1-inch florets (about 6 cups)

1. Preheat the oven to 375°F.
2. Combine everything but the cauliflower in a large bowl. Mix well. Add the cauliflower florets and toss to coat well.
3. Place the coated florets on a nonstick baking sheet in a single layer. Bake for 25 minutes or until golden brown.
4. Toss with extra red hot sauce if desired.

SALADS

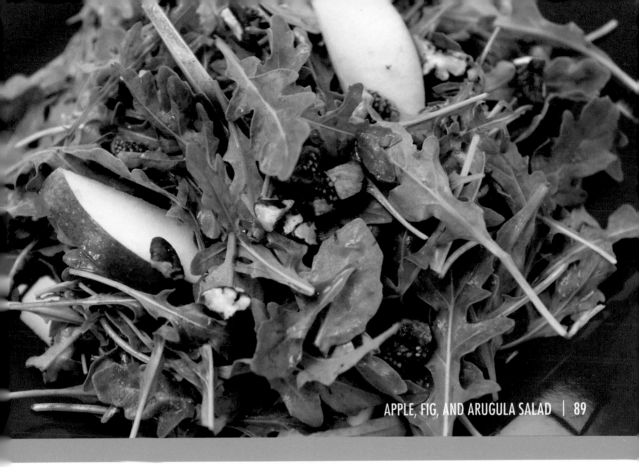

FRESH SPINACH SALAD

MAKES 4 SERVINGS

This salad makes a refreshing side dish to any number of entrées, sandwiches, or soups in this book, and if you keep All-Purpose Vinaigrette on hand, you can have this salad ready in 10 minutes.

2 large bunches spinach, stemmed and thinly sliced (about 8 cups)
1 large red bell pepper, diced
1 bunch green onions, thinly sliced
½ cup All-Purpose Vinaigrette (p. 44), more or less to taste
¼ cup toasted sunflower seeds (optional)

1. Combine all ingredients in a large bowl and toss to mix well.
2. To serve, divide the salad among four plates.

MAKE IT EASY

- You can also buy baby spinach pre-washed in most grocery stores. It will save you the time of washing bunched spinach.
- If the spinach doesn't look good in the store the day you shop, use mixed greens, arugula, or any other light leafy green you can find.

APPLE, FIG, AND ARUGULA SALAD PICTURED ON PAGE 87

MAKES 4 SERVINGS

The peppery arugula, toasted pecans, and tart and sweet fruits in this salad make it a perfect accompaniment for any dish—or a quick, easy meal on its own when cooking seems like too much work.

8 cups arugula
1 large Fuji apple, cored and chopped
6 figs, chopped
½ cup toasted chopped pecans
½ cup All-Purpose Vinaigrette (p. 44)

1. Combine everything in a large bowl and toss to mix well.
2. To serve, divide the salad among four plates.

TIPS

- If you don't like arugula, use spinach or any other light salad green.
- Walnuts work just as well as the pecans. My personal preference is pecans.

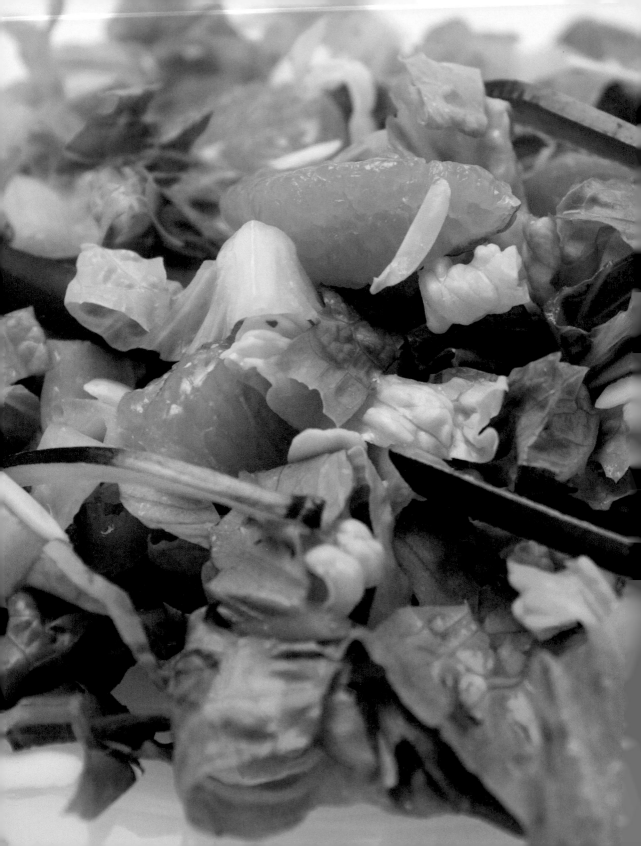

ORANGE-MISO ROMAINE SALAD

MAKES 4 SERVINGS

The hearty romaine lettuce holds up well to the equally hearty Orange-Miso Salad Dressing. I eat this as a side dish, or as an entrée when I want a light, refreshing meal.

1 large head romaine lettuce, coarsely chopped
⅓–½ cup Orange-Miso Salad Dressing (p. 48)
1 navel orange, peeled and sectioned
1 small red onion, thinly sliced
¼ cup toasted slivered almonds

1. Combine the romaine lettuce and Orange-Miso Salad Dressing in a bowl and toss to mix well.
2. Divide the lettuce among four plates and top with the remaining ingredients.

MAKE IT EASY

Buy pre-chopped bagged romaine lettuce and canned mandarin oranges in juice (drain the juice off before adding the oranges to the salad).

KALE SALAD WITH ORANGE-MISO DRESSING

MAKES 4 SERVINGS

The Orange-Miso Salad Dressing and the fresh oranges really mellow out the kale in this salad.

2 large bunches kale, stemmed and coarsely chopped (about 8 cups)
1 15-ounce can cannellini beans, drained and rinsed
¾ cup Orange-Miso Salad Dressing (p. 48), more or less to taste
1 large orange, peeled and sectioned
1 medium red onion, thinly sliced

1. Combine everything in a large bowl and toss to mix well.
2. To serve, divide the salad among four plates.

> **TIP**
>
> I like to let my kale salad sit for an hour to let the salad dressing mellow out the slightly chewy, slightly bitter kale. Alternatively, you can use the less bitter, more tender baby kale greens if you can find them, or spinach if you are in a hurry.

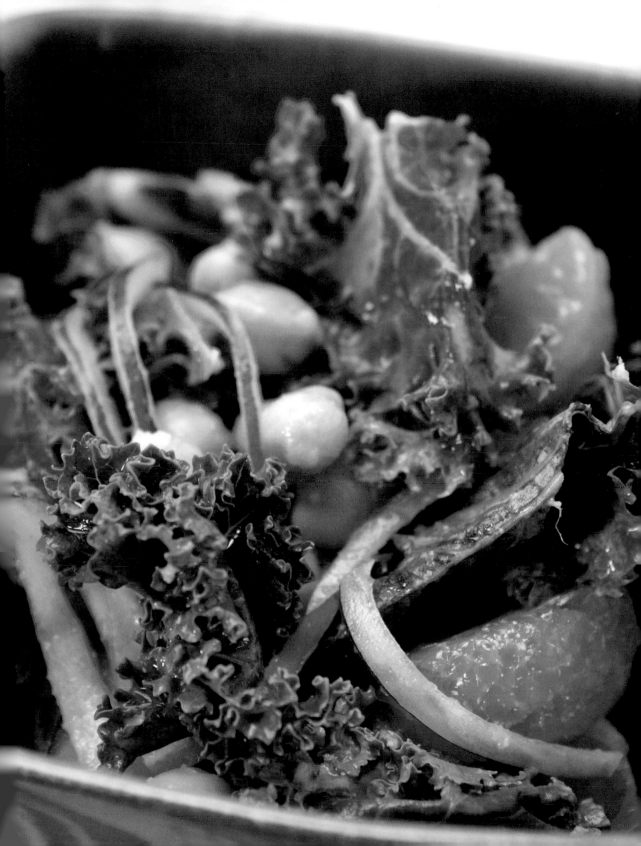

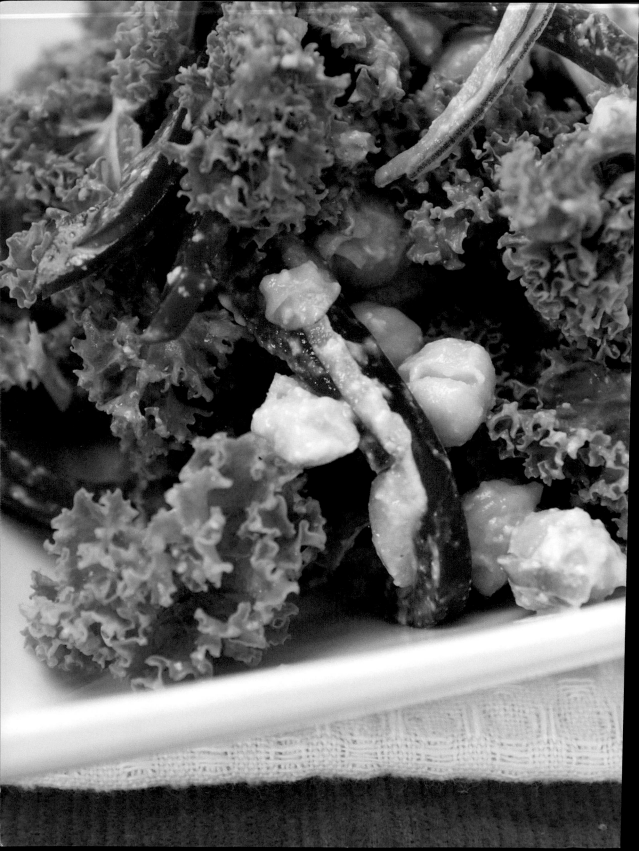

BEAN AND KALE SALAD WITH CREAMY CASHEW-LIME DRESSING

MAKES 4 SERVINGS

The tart and creamy dressing in this salad balances the sometimes bitter kale nicely. Adding beans makes this dish hearty enough for a meal.

¼ cup roasted unsalted cashews
1½ tablespoons mellow white miso paste
¼ cup lime juice
½ teaspoon cayenne pepper (optional)
¼ cup water

2 large bunches kale, stemmed and coarsely chopped (about 8 cups)
1 15-ounce can garbanzo beans (chickpeas), drained and rinsed

1. Combine the cashews, miso, lime juice, cayenne pepper, and water in a blender and puree until smooth and creamy.
2. Add the kale and garbanzo beans to a bowl and add the cashew dressing. Mix well.
3. To serve, divide the salad among four plates.

> **TIP**
>
> I usually like to let this salad sit for an hour before serving it to give the dressing a chance to soften the kale. If you can find baby kale in your grocery store, use it. It's tender and has a milder flavor. You can use raw cashew in the salad dressing, but I like the flavor of toasted nuts more than raw. For a lower-fat version of this salad, use Asian Salad Dressing (p. 45). You'll need about 1 cup of whatever dressing you use.

WARM KALE SALAD WITH PEANUT DRESSING

MAKES 4 SERVINGS

A friend of mine told me once there was no way she would ever get her kids to eat kale. I took that as a dare. I made them this dish and they loved it. For a low-fat warm kale salad, make this dish with Asian Salad Dressing (p. 45).

1 small red onion, thinly sliced
1 medium red bell pepper, diced
¾ cup Almost Instant Peanut Sauce (p. 51)
3 or 4 large bunches kale, stemmed and chopped (about 16 cups)
1 teaspoon crushed red pepper flakes (optional)

1. Combine the red onion and red bell pepper in a large pot and cook over medium heat for 5 minutes.
2. Add the peanut sauce, kale, and crushed red pepper flakes and cook, stirring frequently, until the kale wilts, about 8–9 minutes.

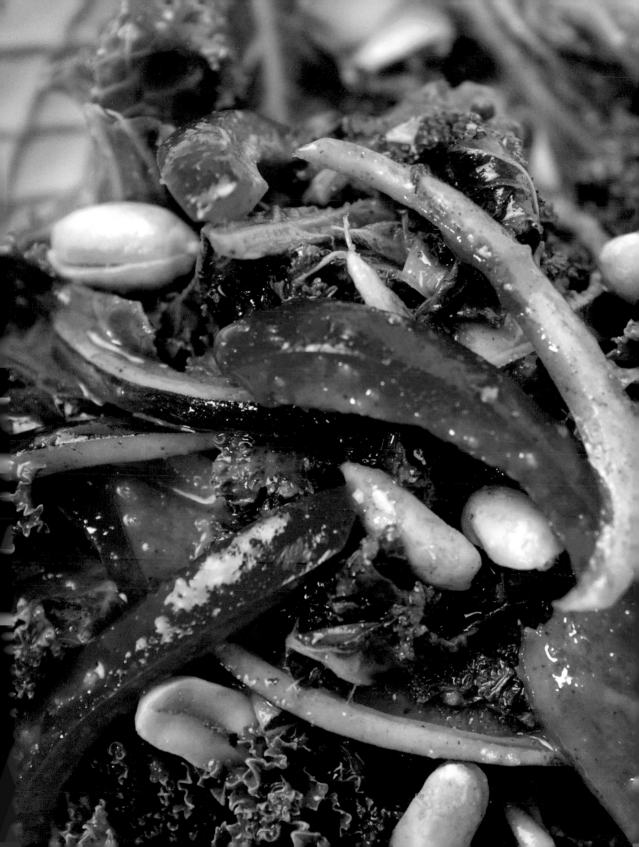

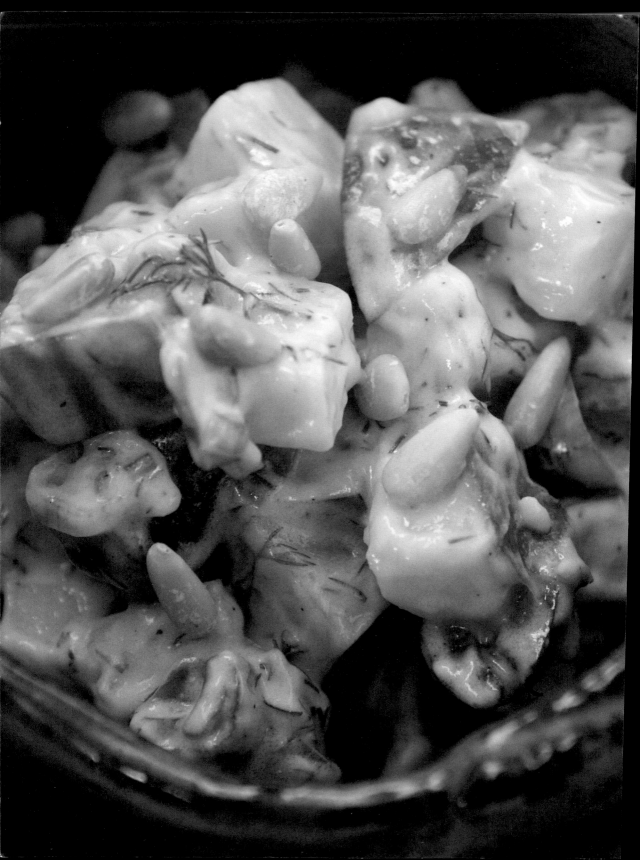

POTATO SALAD WITH PINE NUTS, OLIVES, AND DILL

MAKES 4–6 SERVINGS

I like potato salad but every now and then I like to change it up a little. Pine nuts and olives are not the usual for this salad, but they add a nice Greek flair to this otherwise popular American fare. Serve this on a bed of spinach and you have a good meal.

2 pounds red skin potatoes, cut into ½–inch cubes
1 cup Basic Mayonnaise (p. 53)
4 green onions, sliced
½ cup toasted pine nuts
½ cup pitted kalamata olives
¼ cup minced fresh dill
sea salt and black pepper to taste

1. Place the potatoes in a large pot and cover with 2 quarts of cold salted water.
2. Bring the pot to a boil over medium-high heat. Reduce the heat to medium-low and cook until the potatoes are tender, about 8–10 minutes.
3. When the potatoes are tender, drain them in a colander and rinse under cold water until cool. Drain again and add them to a bowl with the remaining ingredients.
4. Mix well and chill until ready to serve.

LATE SUMMER POTATO–GREEN BEAN SALAD

MAKES 4–6 SERVINGS

I like potato salad made with something besides mayonnaise for a change of pace. It is a little lighter, especially in the heat of summer. You can make this salad any time of year, but green beans are in season in the summer.

1½ pounds red skin potatoes, cut into ½-inch cubes
¾ pound fresh green beans, trimmed and halved
1 red bell pepper, diced small
1 small yellow onion, diced small
½ cup All-Purpose Vinaigrette (p. 44)
1 tablespoon dried tarragon or
    2 tablespoons minced fresh tarragon
sea salt and black pepper to taste

1. In a large pot, bring 2 quarts of water to a boil.
2. Add the potatoes and green beans and cook over medium heat for 7 minutes.
3. Drain and rinse the vegetables under cold water. Add the vegetables to a bowl with the remaining ingredients.
4. Season with salt and pepper. Gently toss to mix well.

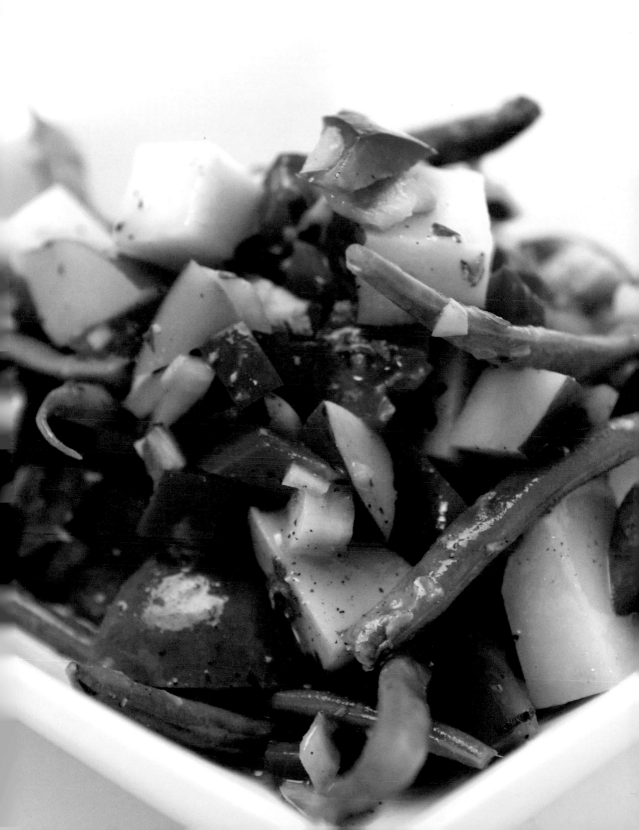

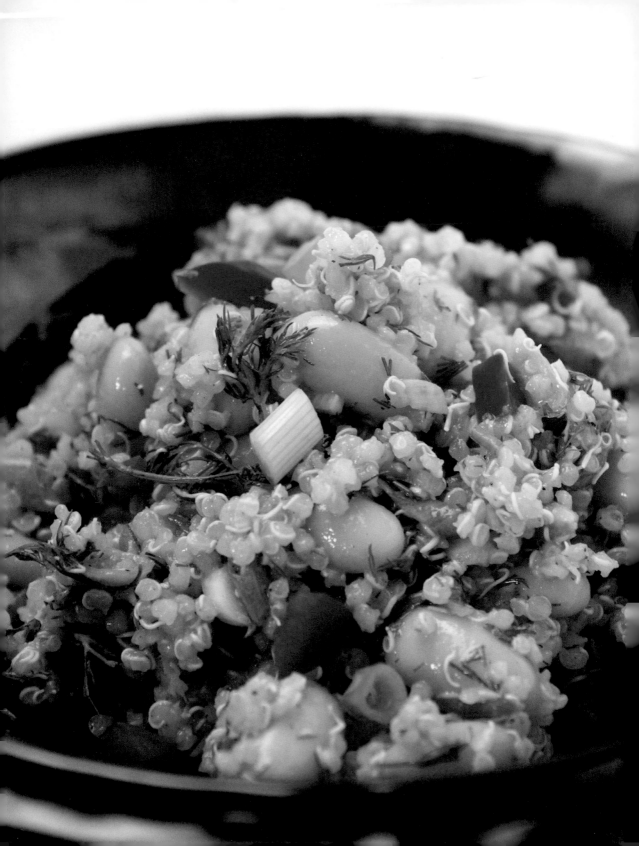

BEANS AND GRAIN SALAD

MAKES 4 SERVINGS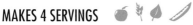

Think of this as your master bean and grain salad recipe. Vary the flavors by using different herbs, vegetables, or even different acids—vinegar, lemon juice, or lime juice. Serve this salad on a bed of greens or wrap it up in a whole grain tortilla with ¼ cup Green Sauce (p. 52) for a meal on the go.

1 15-ounce can beans (black, pinto, navy, red, or white kidney), drained and rinsed
2 cups cooked grains
½ bunch (about 6) green onions, sliced
1 medium red bell pepper (green or poblano will also work)

4–5 tablespoons lemon or lime juice or All-Purpose Vinaigrette (p. 44)
1 cup chopped fresh herbs (basil, cilantro, tarragon, mint, or a combination of any of these)
sea salt and black pepper to taste

1. Combine everything in a bowl and mix well.
2. To serve, divide the salad among four plates. Store refrigerated in an airtight container for up to 4 days.

MAKE IT EASY

- Keep canned beans and cooked brown rice on hand and you can have a meal ready in minutes. I like brown rice but if I forgot to cook it on Sunday, or if I ran out, then quick-cooking grains like quinoa or millet will work just fine.
- For a little kick, add in: 1 seeded and finely diced jalapeno pepper and/or 1 tablespoon toasted ground cumin.

CHICKPEA SALAD WITH SUN-DRIED TOMATO VINAIGRETTE

MAKES 4 SERVINGS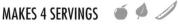

Many versions of this salad call for up to ½ cup olive oil to make the dressing. My version has all the flavor of those fat-laden salads without the oil.

½ cup sun-dried tomato halves (not packed in oil)
3 tablespoons red wine vinegar
2 15-ounce cans garbanzo beans (chickpeas), drained and rinsed
1 15-ounce can artichoke hearts in brine, quartered

1 medium red onion, diced
1 cup fresh basil leaves, chopped
2 tablespoons toasted pine nuts (optional)
sea salt and black pepper to taste
4 cups arugula or other greens

1. Add the sun-dried tomato halves to a small saucepan and add water to cover.
2. Bring the pan to a simmer and cook the sun-dried tomatoes until tender, about 10 minutes.
3. Add the tomatoes to a blender with ½ cup of the cooking water and process until smooth. Add more water if necessary to get a creamy texture. Discard any unused water.
4. Add the mixture to a bowl and add the red wine vinegar, garbanzo beans, artichoke hearts, red onion, basil, and pine nuts.
5. Season with salt and pepper to taste.
6. Divide the arugula among four plates and spoon the chickpea salad evenly over the greens.

MAKE IT EASY

Look for sun-dried tomatoes that are not packed in oil. I buy them in the bulk section of my food co-op fully dried. You'll also find them vacuum packed. If your grocer doesn't carry them you can find them online at many natural foods retailers. Alternatively, you can make this recipe with fresh tomatoes, or canned: you will need about 1 cup diced, plus an extra tablespoon of red wine vinegar.

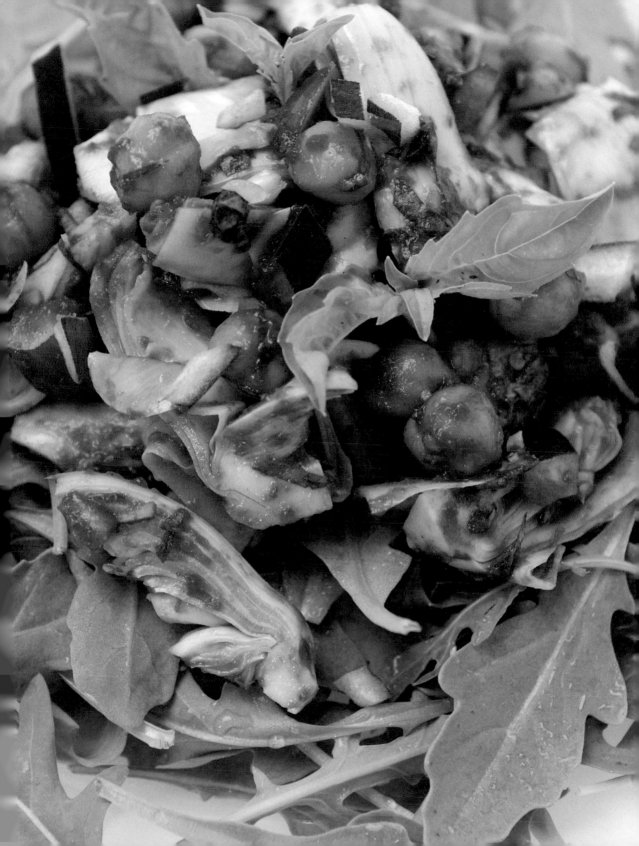

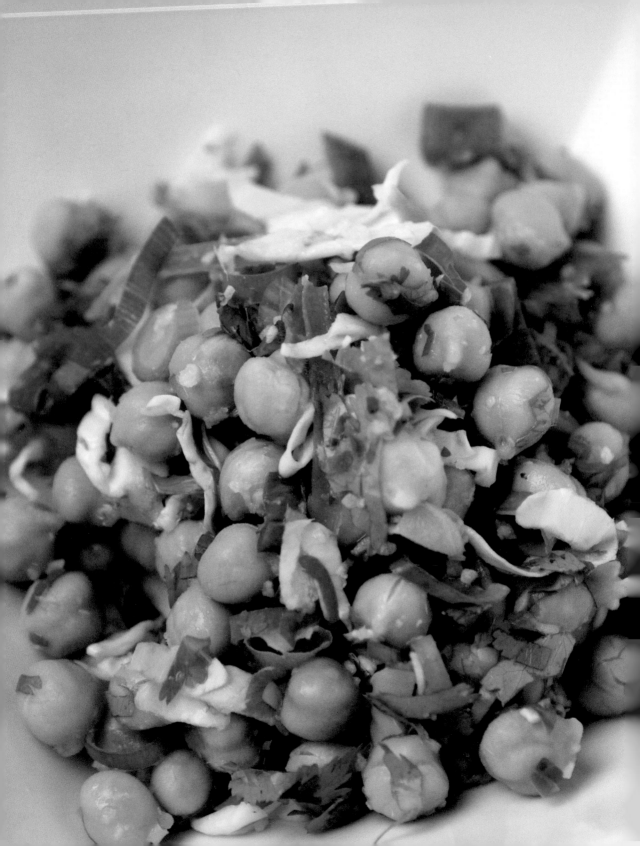

ASIAN CHICKPEA SALAD

MAKES 6 SERVINGS

This is one of my favorite meals, especially when I don't want to turn the stove on or when I'm going on a road trip and want to make sure I have something healthy to eat with me. I always keep the Basic Mayonnaise recipe on hand so I can have quick, flavorful foods like this around. I eat this salad in pita bread with sprouts or on toast with a tomato slice.

**1 15-ounce can garbanzo beans (chickpeas),
    drained, rinsed, and lightly mashed
1 carrot, grated
½ cup Basic Mayonnaise (p. 53)
¼ cup chopped fresh cilantro
¼ cup toasted cashews
4 green onions, sliced
2 teaspoons low-sodium soy sauce or tamari
1 teaspoon grated ginger**

1   Add everything to a bowl and mix well.

FANCY-PANTS CHICKPEA SALAD

MAKES 7 SERVINGS

This is my mock tuna salad for grown-ups—although I have served it to kids who like this version too. I eat it with rice crackers or on a whole wheat bun with sprouts or lettuce.

2 15-ounce cans garbanzo beans (chickpeas),
   drained, rinsed, and lightly mashed
1 cup Basic Mayonnaise (p. 53)
½ cup toasted slivered almonds (optional)
½ cup dill pickle relish
¼ cup capers, drained (optional)
1 tablespoon fresh chopped dill
sea salt and black pepper to taste

1. Combine everything in a large bowl and mix well. Store refrigerated in an airtight container for up to 4 days.

ORANGE, BEAN, AND OLIVE SALAD

MAKES 7 SERVINGS

I make this easy salad all summer long and often I serve it in a wrap with hummus. Take this to your next picnic as a change from the usual picnic fare.

2 15-ounce cans cannellini beans, drained and rinsed
2 large oranges, peeled and cut into segments
½ medium red onion, diced small
½ cup pitted kalamata olives
½ cup Herbed Orange Vinaigrette (p. 47)
sea salt and crushed red pepper flakes to taste
4 cups fresh spinach or your favorite greens

1. Combine all ingredients except for spinach in a large bowl and mix well.
2. Serve on a bed of fresh spinach or your favorite greens.

BLACK-EYED PEA SALAD

MAKES 4 SERVINGS

This salad works well with any of the vinaigrettes in this cookbook, such as the Asian Salad Dressing (p. 45), the Herbed Orange Vinaigrette (p. 47), or the All-Purpose Vinaigrette. It is another one of those salads I like to make when there is basil in the garden and tomatoes are perfectly ripe.

3 15-ounce cans black-eyed peas, drained and rinsed
4 cloves garlic, minced
6 green onions, sliced
1 large ripe tomato, chopped
1 cup chopped fresh basil
½ cup All-Purpose Vinaigrette (p. 44), more or less to taste
sea salt and black pepper to taste

1. Combine all ingredients in a bowl; let sit in the refrigerator for a couple of hours to blend flavors.

BARLEY SALAD WITH APPLES AND WALNUTS

MAKES 4 SERVINGS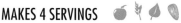

This salad is bright with flavor and it is filling when made with hearty barley. But you can also use whatever grain you have on hand to make this dish. It is a perfect late-summer meal.

1 cup barley
2½ cups water
2 Fuji apples, cored and diced
1 stalk celery
2 tablespoons chopped fresh tarragon
½ cup toasted chopped walnuts (optional)
½ cup All-Purpose Vinaigrette (p. 44), more or less to taste
sea salt and black pepper to taste

1. Combine the barley and water in a small saucepan.
2. Bring the pan to a boil over high heat, then reduce the heat to medium, cover, and cook the barley for 45 minutes.
3. Rinse the barley to cool. Combine it with the remaining ingredients in a bowl and mix well. Refrigerate until ready to serve.

GREEN SESAME PASTA SALAD

MAKES 4–6 SERVINGS

Cilantro and tahini seem made for each other and they come together nicely in this pasta salad. The arugula adds a nice peppery bite, but you can use spinach if you prefer.

1 12-ounce package whole grain fusilli or
   other tube-shaped pasta
1 cup Green Sauce (p. 52)
3 cups arugula
1 medium red bell pepper, diced
4 green onions, thinly sliced
sea salt and black pepper to taste

1. Cook the pasta according to package instructions. Drain and rinse until cooled.
2. Combine all ingredients in a large bowl and mix well.

RED PEPPER SLAW

MAKES 6 SERVINGS

I like coleslaw but rarely want the traditional mayonnaise-laden version unless it is Red Pepper Mayo. The roasted red bell peppers make a bright, beautiful slaw to look at, and the flavor is a perfect contrast to earthy dishes like Portobello Mushroom Burgers (p. 124).

¾ **cup Red Pepper Mayo (p. 54), more or less to taste**
1 pound slaw mix (about 7 cups)
2 tablespoons chopped fresh dill
black pepper to taste

1. Combine everything in a bowl and toss to mix well.
2. To serve, divide the salad among six plates. Store refrigerated in an airtight container for up to 2 days.

PEANUT SLAW

MAKES 4 SERVINGS

Peanut Slaw is a great twist on traditional coleslaw, which I love but get a little bored with. This lighter version uses a vinaigrette instead of the usual mayonnaise and is just as versatile. I eat it with Mushroom Tacos (p. 206) and Portobello Mushroom Burgers (p. 124). It's also great as a side dish to take to picnics.

6 cups slaw mix
¾ cup Asian Salad Dressing (p. 45)
6 green onions, chopped
½ cup toasted peanuts

1. Combine everything in a bowl and toss to mix well. Store refrigerated in an airtight container for up to 5 days.

> **TIP**
>
> Try some of the fun variations on slaw mixes in your grocery store, like broccoli slaw or angel hair slaw for a change.

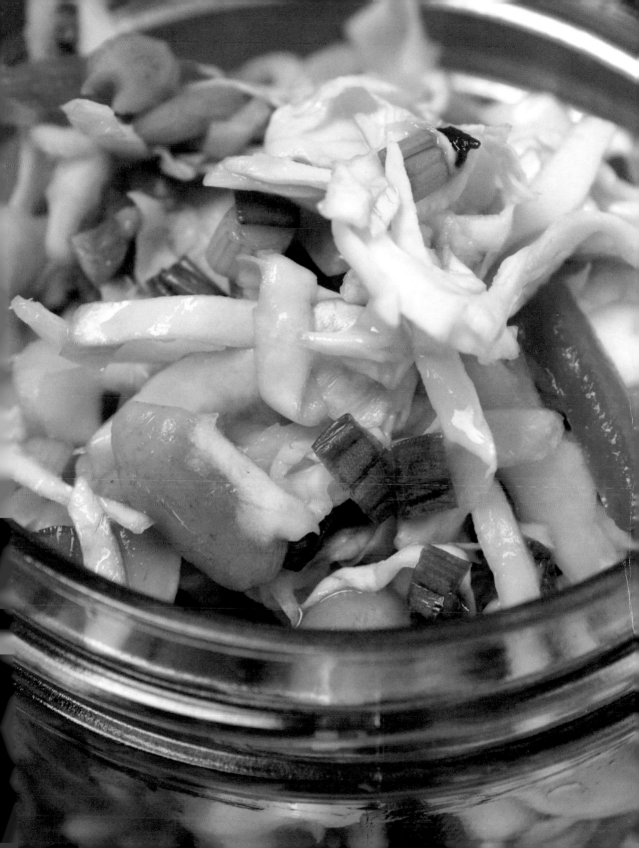

SANDWICHES

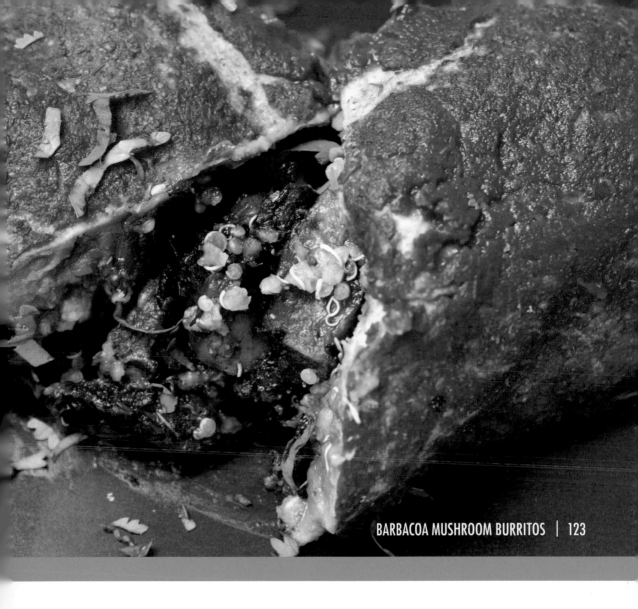

BARBACOA MUSHROOM BURRITOS | 123

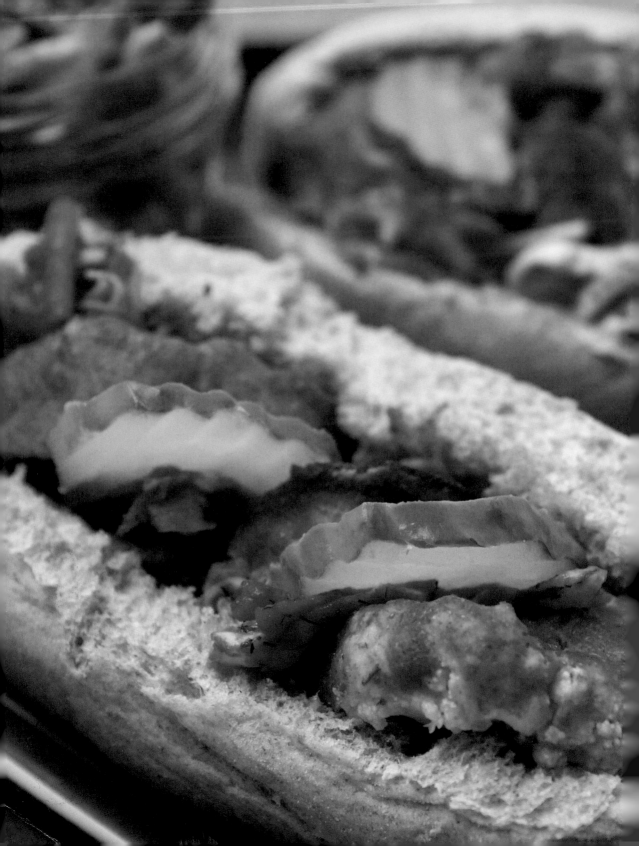

BUFFALO PO' BOYS

MAKES 4 PO' BOYS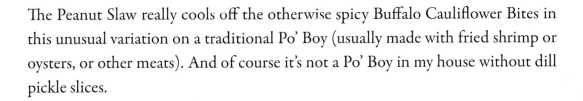

The Peanut Slaw really cools off the otherwise spicy Buffalo Cauliflower Bites in this unusual variation on a traditional Po' Boy (usually made with fried shrimp or oysters, or other meats). And of course it's not a Po' Boy in my house without dill pickle slices.

4 hoagie buns
1 recipe Buffalo Cauliflower Bites (p. 85)
1 recipe Peanut Slaw (p. 114)
dill pickle slices
1 small red onion, thinly sliced

1. Slice the hoagie buns in half lengthwise.
2. Place the cauliflower bites over the bottom half of the buns.
3. Spoon some of the Peanut Slaw over the cauliflower, then top with the pickle slices, red onion slices, and finally the top half of the hoagie bun. Serve immediately.

PULLED MUSHROOM SANDWICHES

MAKES 4 SANDWICHES

A popular foodie idea is the concept of pulled pork or pulled chicken or pulled whatever. I like barbecue sandwiches as much as the next person, but I don't want the unhealthy meat in my diet. I do want to go to a cookout and have a great sandwich, however. Mine just happens to be healthy.

1 medium yellow onion, thinly sliced
1 pound portobello mushrooms, cut into thin strips
½ cup Easy Date Barbecue Sauce (p. 59), more or less to taste
4 whole grain sandwich buns, split
1 recipe Peanut Slaw (p. 114)

1. Preheat a medium skillet over medium heat.
2. Add the onions and mushrooms and sauté for 5 minutes, until the onions start to brown and turn translucent.
3. Add the barbecue sauce and cook for 3 minutes.
4. To serve, place the bottom half of each bun on a plate. Divide the mushroom mixture among the four buns. Top with the Peanut Slaw and the top halves of the buns.

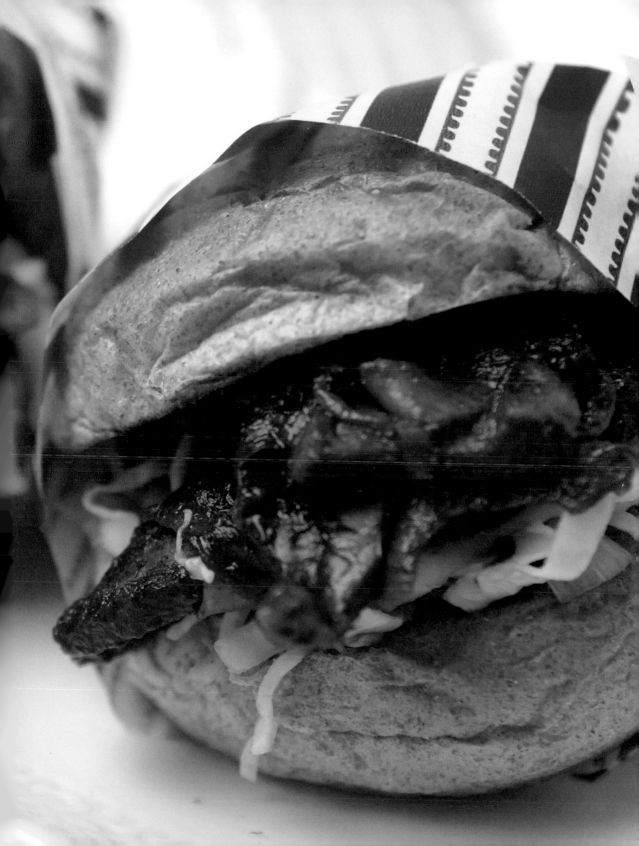

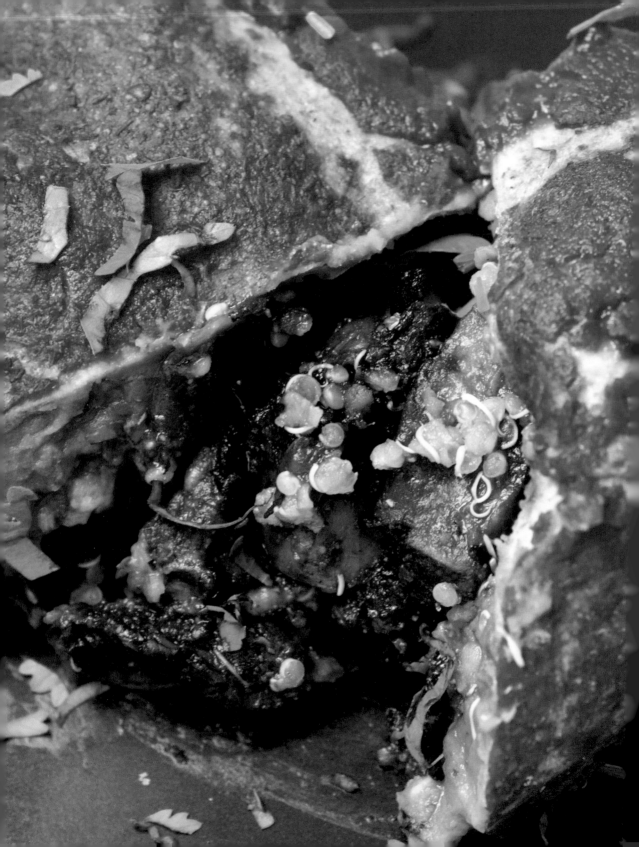

BARBACOA MUSHROOM BURRITOS

MAKES 4 BURRITOS

These burritos are filling and full of flavor. The Mushrooms Barbacoa comes together quickly and if you don't have rice cooked, you can cook quinoa or millet in 15–20 minutes. I make a double batch of the Mushrooms Barbacoa so I can make these burritos one night and Mushroom Tacos (p. 206) another.

4 12-inch whole grain tortillas
1 cup refried beans
2 cups cooked brown rice or quinoa
½ recipe Mushrooms Barbacoa (p. 196)
1 15-ounce can enchilada sauce or
2 cups No-Queso Sauce (p. 67)

1. Preheat the oven to 375°F.
2. Lay the tortillas flat on a work surface. Divide the refried beans among the four tortillas, spreading them over the bottom half of each tortilla.
3. Place ½ cup of the cooked brown rice or quinoa over the refried beans and top with the Mushrooms Barbacoa. Fold the tortillas in over the filling and roll them up.
4. Place the burritos in a baking dish and pour enchilada sauce or No-Queso Sauce over each.
5. Bake for 15 minutes, until the sauce is bubbly.

MAKE IT EASY

If you don't have enchilada sauce or No-Queso Sauce on hand, use your favorite salsa.

PORTOBELLO MUSHROOM BURGERS

MAKES 4 BURGERS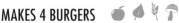

One of the things you can count on in many mainstream restaurants is that if they have a vegan option on the menu, it is often some kind of veggie burger—and half of the time, it is a portobello mushroom burger. Most of the better restaurants know that what makes a good burger is the toppings. I like all kinds of toppings on my burger, such as Red Pepper Slaw (p. 113), Peanut Slaw (p. 114), and even baked beans (try the Jerk-Style Beans [p. 188] and see what I mean). Go wild with your favorite toppings on this burger or go simple—sometimes ketchup and mustard are all you need.

4 portobello mushroom caps
3 tablespoons balsamic vinegar
1 tablespoon low-sodium soy sauce or tamari
3 cloves garlic, minced
2 teaspoons dried basil
1 teaspoon dried oregano
½ teaspoon black pepper

4 whole grain burger buns, toasted
1 large tomato, sliced
4 lettuce leaves
1 small red onion, thinly sliced
½ cup Red Pepper Mayo (p. 54) or your favorite condiments (ketchup, mustard, etc.)

1. Place the mushrooms stem-side up on a nonstick baking sheet.
2. Combine the balsamic vinegar, soy sauce or tamari, garlic, basil, oregano, and black pepper in a small bowl and mix well.
3. Drizzle the marinade over the mushroom caps and let sit for 30 minutes.
4. Preheat the oven to 425°F.
5. Bake the mushrooms for 10 minutes, then turn them over and bake for another 10 minutes.
6. Place each mushroom on the bottom half of a toasted bun and top with the tomato, lettuce, onion slices, and Red Pepper Mayo or condiment of your choice.

VARIATION

Serve topped with Peanut Slaw instead of the lettuce, red onion, and condiments.

SOUTHWEST BURGERS

MAKES 4 BURGERS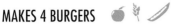

I rarely ever buy packaged veggie burgers at the store. They usually have too much added fat and not much flavor. Why would I go for store-bought when I can make these flavor-packed burgers in less than 30 minutes?

1 cup water
½ cup bulgur
1 cup canned fat-free refried beans
1 tablespoon granulated onion
3 tablespoons arrowroot powder
1½ tablespoons low-sodium soy sauce or tamari

1 tablespoon ground cumin
3–4 tablespoons cornmeal, for baking
4 whole grain burger buns, toasted
1 cup salsa
1 small red onion, sliced
1 avocado, sliced

1. Bring the water to a boil in a small pot and add the bulgur. Bring the pot back to a boil, turn the heat off, and cover the pot with a tight-fitting lid. Let it sit for 10 minutes or until the bulgur is tender and all of the water is absorbed.

2. Add the bulgur to a bowl with beans, granulated onion, arrowroot powder, soy sauce or tamari, and cumin and mix well.

3. Divide the burger mixture into four equal parts and shape each part into a ball. Dredge the balls in the cornmeal, shake off the excess, and press them flat into patties.

4. Cook the burgers in a nonstick skillet for 5 minutes over medium heat, turn them over, and cook them for 5 minutes more. Alternatively, preheat the oven to 350°F. Bake the burgers on a nonstick baking sheet for 20 minutes. Turn them over gently and bake for another 15 minutes.

5. Place each patty on the bottom half of a toasted bun and top with the salsa, onion, and avocado.

VARIATION

Use Fresh Herbed Tomato-Corn Salsa (p. 58) as a condiment.

WARM MUSHROOM SALAD SANDWICHES

MAKES 4 SANDWICHES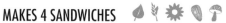

A friend of mine used to make this sandwich as a late-night snack using leftover sauce she had from pasta. I fell in love with it and asked her often where the idea came from to make this delicious sauce into a sandwich—she never told me. This is my interpretation of that late-night snack. I eat it frequently, sometimes on toasted bread, open faced, and sometimes on a bun.

1 medium onion, chopped
1 pound cremini mushrooms
2 teaspoons chopped fresh dill
sea salt and black pepper to taste
1 cup Mori-Nu Silken Lite Firm Tofu or Cauliflower Puree (p. 64)
2 tablespoons toasted pine nuts
1 teaspoon freshly squeezed lemon juice
4 lettuce leaves
4 whole grain sandwich buns

1. Heat a skillet over medium-high heat.

2. Add the onion and mushrooms and sauté for 5 minutes. Add 1–2 tablespoons of water as needed to keep the vegetables from sticking to the pan.

3. Add the fresh dill, season with sea salt and black pepper, and set aside.

4. In a blender, combine the silken tofu or Cauliflower Puree, pine nuts, lemon juice, and a pinch of salt and pepper and puree until smooth and creamy.

5. Add the tofu mixture to the pan with the mushrooms and mix well.

6. Place lettuce leaves on the bottom half of each sandwich bun and top with the mushroom mixture. Top with the other half of the bun.

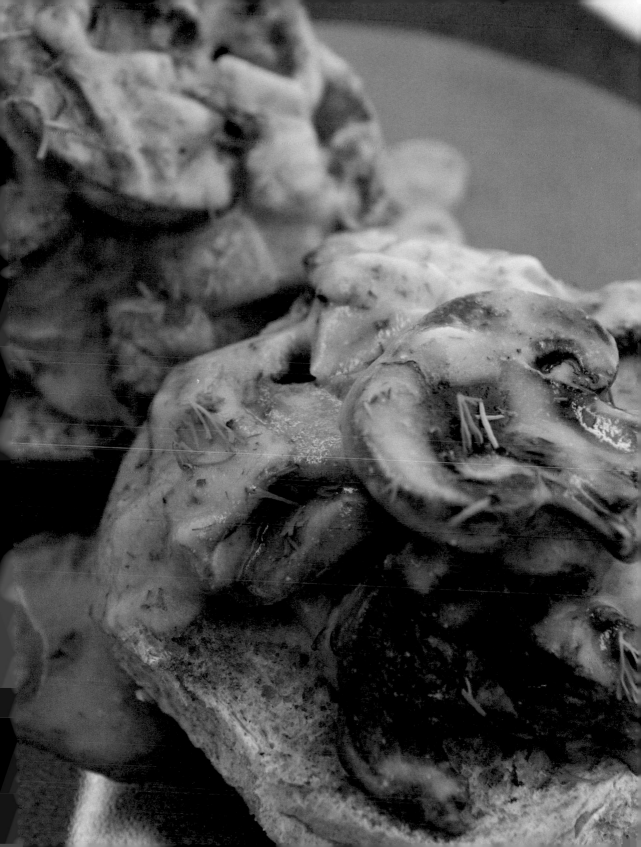

PASTA & BAKED DISHES

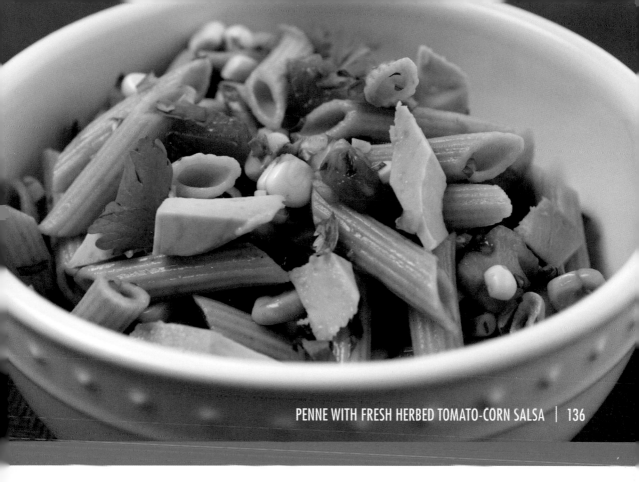

CHILLED PEANUT NOODLES

MAKES 4–6 SERVINGS

I love anything with peanut butter—especially a spoon. I only eat peanut butter as a special treat because of the fat content, and this dish is one of my favorite special treats. This dish, like Almond Noodles (p. 133), comes together quickly. If you are cooking for one or two, you can put as much pasta as you want in a bowl, toss it with an appropriate amount of sauce, and save the rest of the sauce for use with the Quinoa–Black Bean Buddha Bowl (p. 201) or Thai Pita Pizza (p. 211).

1 pound whole grain spaghetti
½–¾ cup Almost Instant Peanut Sauce (p. 51)
1 cup chopped fresh green onion
chopped peanuts for garnish

1. Cook the spaghetti according to package instructions.
2. Drain the noodles, rinse under cold water, and drain again.
3. Add the cooked spaghetti to a bowl with the peanut sauce and toss to mix well.
4. Serve garnished with the chopped green onion and chopped peanuts.

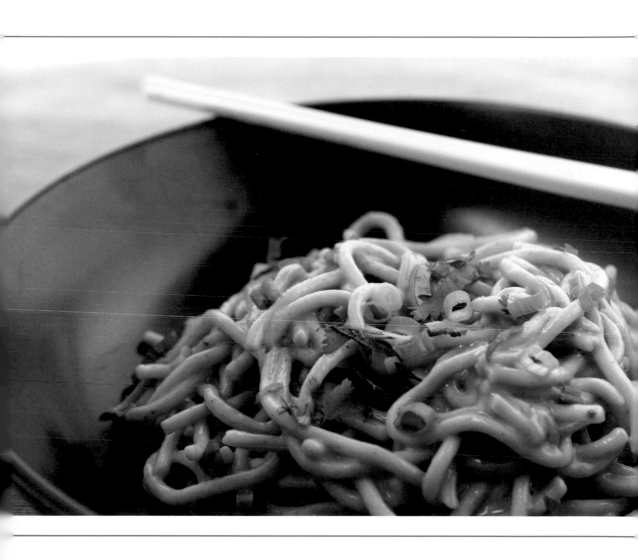

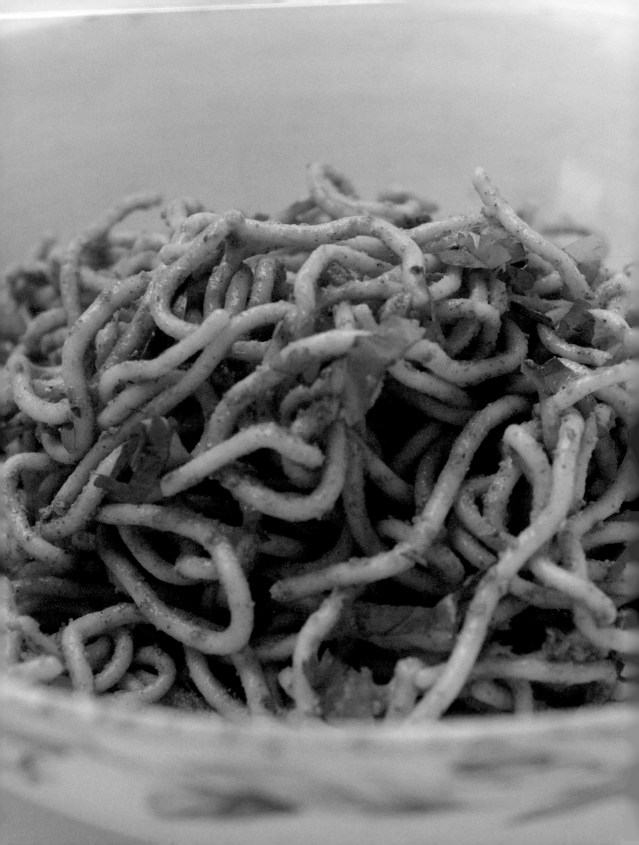

ALMOND NOODLES

MAKES 6 SERVINGS

The rich sauce for this flavorful treat comes together even before you finish cooking the pasta. I make this dish when I need to have dinner on the table in a hurry, and, if I planned my week right, I already have cooked pasta in the refrigerator, so I can have a meal ready in less than 15 minutes.

1 pound whole grain spaghetti
½ cup almond butter
¼ cup water
¼ cup rice wine vinegar
2 tablespoons low-sodium soy sauce or tamari
2 tablespoons Thai red curry paste
chopped fresh cilantro for garnish

1. Cook the spaghetti according to package instructions.
2. While the spaghetti cooks, combine the almond butter, water, rice vinegar, soy sauce or tamari, and Thai red curry paste in a large bowl and whisk together.
3. Add the cooked spaghetti to the sauce and toss to mix well.
4. Serve garnished with the chopped cilantro.

ORANGE-MISO NOODLES

I eat this dish a lot in the summer. It is light, refreshing, and yummy.

12 ounces whole grain noodles
Orange-Miso Salad Dressing (p. 48)
4 green onions, thinly sliced
½ cup chopped fresh cilantro

1. Cook the noodles according to package instructions, then rinse them until completely cooled to stop their cooking.

2. Add the cooled noodles to a bowl with the remaining ingredients. Mix well.

3. To serve, divide the noodles among four plates.

VARIATION

Make a double batch of the dressing and serve this recipe on a bed of spinach. You will need 1 cup of greens per serving, tossed with dressing to taste. Place the greens on a plate and then top with the noodle salad.

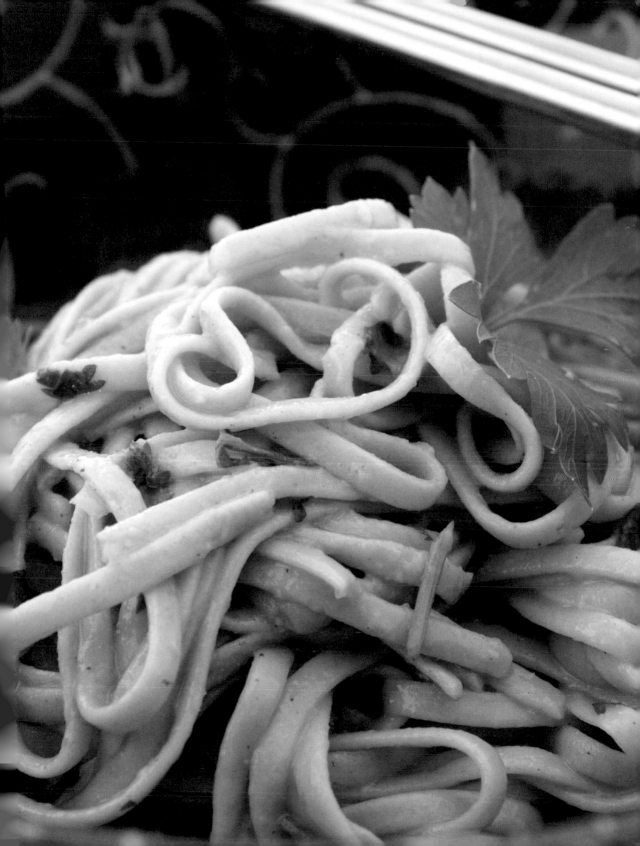

PENNE WITH FRESH HERBED TOMATO-CORN SALSA

PICTURED ON PAGE 129

MAKES 4 SERVINGS

I gravitate to this recipe every summer when tomatoes and corn are fresh and ripe in the garden. The avocado makes it creamy, but if you want a lower-fat dish, you can leave it out.

12 ounces whole grain penne
Fresh Herbed Tomato-Corn Salsa (p. 58)
1 ripe avocado, diced

1. Cook the pasta according to package instructions.
2. Drain and add to a bowl with the remaining ingredients. Mix well.

MAKE IT EASY

Make a double batch of the Fresh Herbed Tomato-Corn Salsa and use the extra for Tostadas (p. 207), or even as a condiment for Southwest Burgers (p. 125).

MOROCCAN PASTA SALAD WITH WHITE BEANS AND SUN-DRIED TOMATOES

MAKES 4 SERVINGS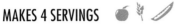

Basil, mint, and cilantro are everywhere in Moroccan food. I sometimes use them all in this dish, making it full flavored and vibrant.

12 ounces whole grain rotini

12 sun-dried tomato halves (not packed in oil), cut into thin strips

1 15-ounce can cannellini beans, drained and rinsed

½ cup finely chopped fresh cilantro or basil

1 tablespoon minced fresh mint

2 teaspoons ground cumin

5 tablespoons lemon juice or balsamic vinegar

2 cloves garlic, minced

sea salt and black pepper to taste

1. Bring a large pot of water to a boil.

2. Add the pasta and cook according to package instructions, adding the sun-dried tomatoes in the last 5 minutes of cooking. Drain and rinse until cooled to room temperature.

3. Place the pasta and sun-dried tomatoes in a large bowl and add the beans, cilantro, mint, cumin, lemon juice, and garlic. Season with sea salt and black pepper to taste.

4. Refrigerate for 1 hour to allow the flavors to marry before serving.

> **TIP**
>
> If you are not a fan of mint, you can leave it out of this recipe. Use fresh, not bottled lemon juice. It makes all the difference in the flavor. You can also use fresh tomatoes in place of the sun-dried tomatoes, if they are in season.

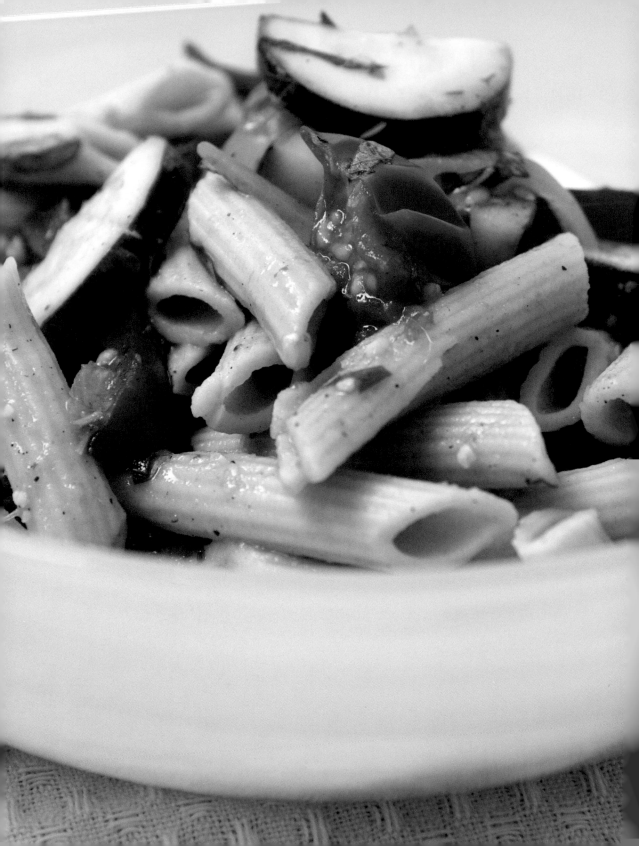

SUMMER PENNE PASTA SAUTÉ

MAKES 4–6 SERVINGS

Everywhere I go people try to give me their extra tomatoes, zucchini, and basil from their garden. I always say yes to the zucchini, but I have more basil than I can use from my own garden. I use these ingredients in any number of dishes, but inevitably they end up in this recipe as well.

1 medium yellow onion, thinly sliced
1 large red bell pepper, cut into 1-inch cubes
1 large zucchini, cut in half lengthwise and
    thinly sliced
1 pint cherry tomatoes, halved

4 cloves garlic, minced
12 large basil leaves, torn
12 ounces whole grain penne
sea salt and black pepper to taste

1. Cook the pasta according to package instructions, reserving 1 cup of the cooking liquid before draining it.

2. Sauté the onion and red bell pepper for 5 minutes over medium-high heat. Add water 1–2 tablespoons at a time to keep the vegetables from sticking.

3. Add the zucchini and cherry tomatoes, and cook for 3 minutes more.

4. Add the garlic, basil, and pasta cooking water, and cook for another minute.

5. Add the cooked pasta and season with salt and pepper. Mix well.

> **MAKE IT EASY**
>
> Use whatever vegetable you want for this dish, but remember that some vegetables take longer to cook than others, so you will want to cook those first and then add the quicker-cooking vegetables. If you want to use a bag of frozen vegetables instead of the zucchini, red bell pepper, and cherry tomatoes, add them after you have cooked the onion for 5 minutes, and remember not to overcook them (frozen vegetables are usually partially cooked and only need about 5 minutes of cooking).

PENNE WITH RED LENTILS AND CHARD

MAKES 4 SERVINGS

Quick-cooking red lentils have a creamy texture and savory taste without much effort. They go well with the mild-flavored chard—also a quick cooker. Make this dish with quick-cooking spinach or arugula for a change. The arugula adds a nice peppery bite.

4 cups vegetable stock
1 cup red lentils
3 cloves garlic, minced
1 teaspoon dried thyme
12 ounces whole grain penne
1 large bunch chard, chopped
sea salt and black pepper to taste

1. Combine the vegetable stock, red lentils, garlic, and thyme in a large saucepan and bring to a boil over high heat. Reduce the heat to medium-low and cook the lentils for 20 minutes or until they are tender.

2. While the lentils are cooking, bring a large pot of salted water to a boil and add the penne. Cook according to package instructions. Drain and set aside while you finish the sauce.

3. When the lentils are tender, add the chard and cook for another 5 minutes.

4. Add the cooked pasta to the pan and season with salt and pepper to taste.

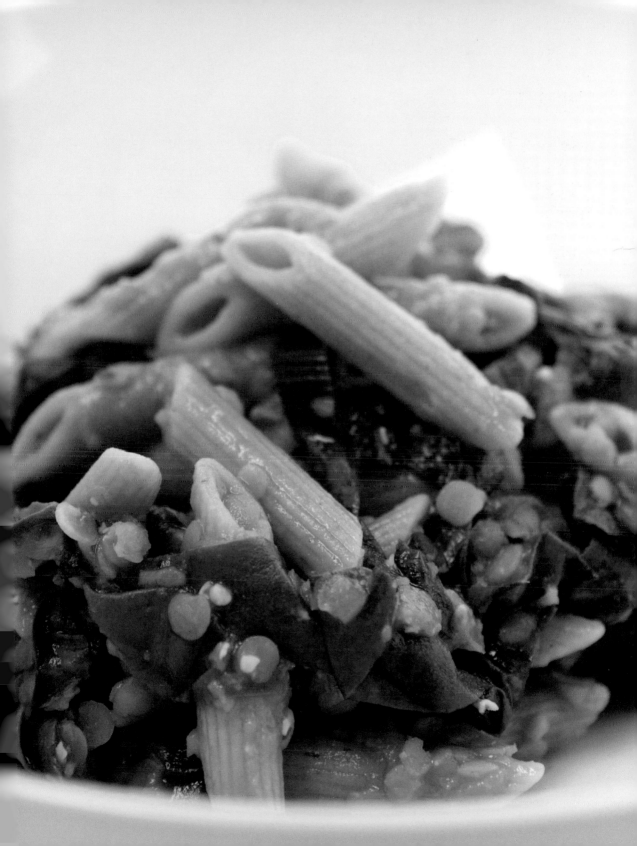

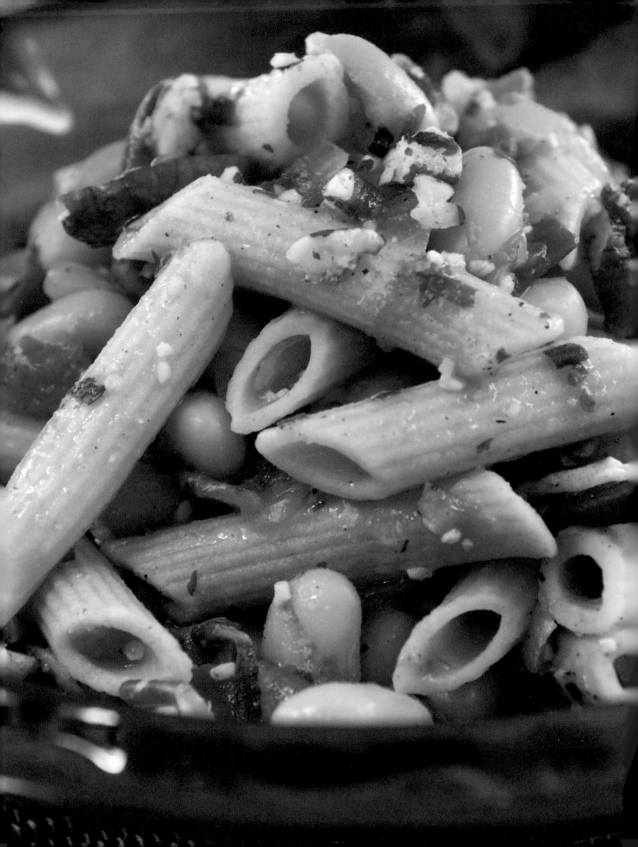

PASTA WITH WHITE BEANS, PECANS, AND TARRAGON

MAKES 4 SERVINGS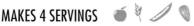

Tarragon, one of my favorite herbs with an almost licorice-like flavor, goes nicely with the earthy sweet toasted pecan. I am always looking for ways to combine the two flavors. But other nuts like walnuts or cashews work too.

12 ounces whole grain penne
1 medium yellow onion, diced
4 cloves garlic, minced
¼ cup fresh tarragon, chopped
1 large tomato, diced

1 15-ounce can cannellini beans,
    drained and rinsed
sea salt and black pepper to taste
½ cup toasted chopped pecans

1. Cook the pasta according to package instructions, reserving 1 cup of the cooking liquid before draining it.

2. While the pasta cooks, sauté the onion in a large saucepan over medium heat for 8 minutes. Add water, 1–2 tablespoons at a time, as needed, to keep the onions from sticking.

3. Add the garlic and cook for another minute. Add the tarragon, tomato, cannellini beans, and some of the pasta cooking liquid. Season with sea salt and black pepper and cook for 5 minutes.

4. Add the cooked pasta and enough of the remaining pasta cooking liquid to make a sauce. Cook for 1 minute to allow the sauce to thicken a little.

5. Serve garnished with the chopped pecans.

> **TIP**
>
> If you want to leave the nuts out to reduce the fat, cook the onions with a package of sliced mushrooms instead and continue with the recipe as written.

PASTA WITH VEGETABLES AND WHITE BEAN–MISO SPREAD

MAKES 6 SERVINGS

Using a bean spread for a sauce is unusual, but it works well when you thin the sauce with a little vegetable stock, and it tastes great.

1 pound whole grain penne
1 12-ounce package frozen mixed vegetables (about 3 cups)
1 recipe White Bean–Miso Spread (p. 77)
low-sodium vegetable stock to taste
1–2 teaspoons crushed red pepper flakes, more or less to taste
8 green onions, thinly sliced

1. Cook the pasta according to package instructions, adding the frozen vegetables to the pot with the pasta in the last 5 minutes of cooking.

2. While the pasta cooks, heat the White Bean–Miso Spread in a large saucepan over medium heat, stirring frequently. Thin the spread with a little vegetable stock to desired sauce consistency.

3. When the pasta and vegetables have finished cooking, drain them and add them to the sauce and mix well.

4. Serve garnished with red pepper flakes and the sliced green onions.

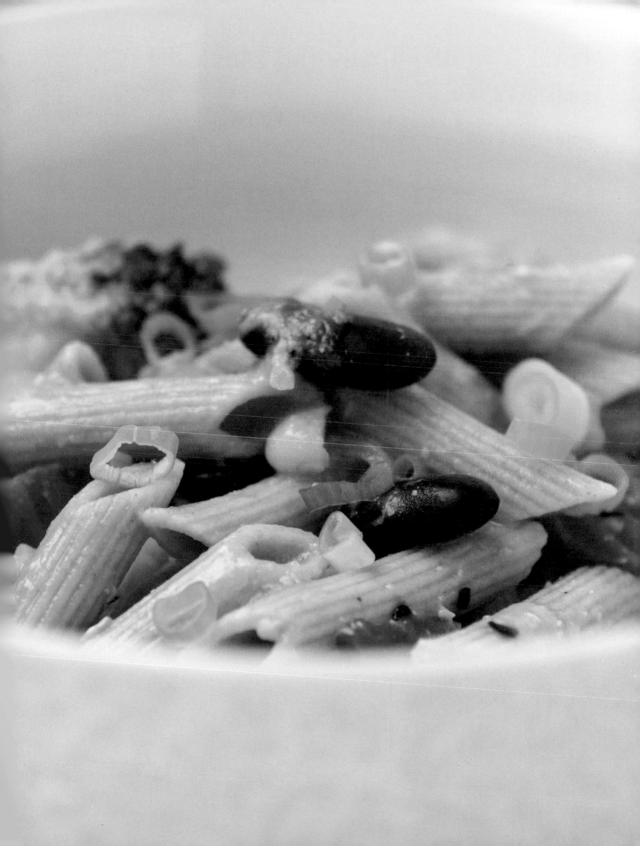

PENNE WITH THAI TOMATO-EGGPLANT SAUCE

MAKES 6 SERVINGS

I think of this sauce as a Thai ratatouille, a stewed eggplant dish popular in parts of the United States and parts of the Mediterranean, especially in the summer. The ginger, red curry paste, and coconut milk are classic Thai ingredients, but if you leave them out and add some fresh basil and chopped zucchini, you would have ratatouille.

1 pound whole grain penne
1 medium yellow onion, diced
1 large eggplant, cut into ½-inch cubes
4 large ripe tomatoes, diced
1 tablespoon minced ginger

4 tablespoons Thai red curry paste
1 14-ounce can light coconut milk
sea salt and black pepper to taste
1 cup cilantro leaves, chopped

1. Bring a large pot of water to a boil. Add the pasta to the boiling water and cook according to package instructions. Drain but do not rinse.

2. Sauté the onion in a large saucepan over medium-high heat for 5 minutes. Add water 1–2 tablespoons at a time to keep the onion from sticking.

3. Add the eggplant and tomatoes and cook for 10 minutes. Add water 1–2 tablespoons at a time as needed to keep the vegetables from sticking to the pan.

4. Add the ginger, Thai red curry paste, and coconut milk to the pan with the vegetables.

5. Mix well and let simmer for 5 minutes. Add the cooked pasta, season with salt and pepper, and cook for 2 minutes to marry the flavors.

6. Serve garnished with the chopped cilantro.

PASTA WITH SAFFRON CREAM

MAKES 4 SERVINGS

I make this dish often for guests. They feel as if they are being treated to something special, and I don't feel as if I spent all day in the kitchen.

12 ounces whole grain rotini
1½ cups frozen peas

1 recipe Saffron Cream (p. 65)
sea salt and black pepper to taste

1. Cook the pasta according to package instructions. Add the frozen peas in the last 4 minutes of cooking.

2. While the pasta cooks, heat the Saffron Cream in a large saucepan (if made ahead of time and cooled).

3. When the pasta and peas have finished cooking, drain them and add them to the pan, letting it simmer for a few minutes.

4. Add sea salt and black pepper to taste.

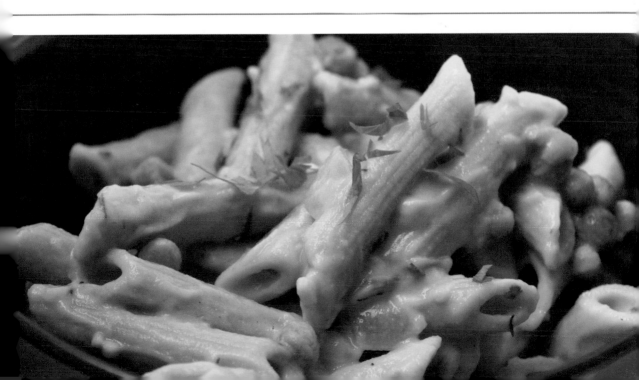

PENNE WITH MUSHROOM-DILL CREAM SAUCE

MAKES 4–6 SERVINGS

This creamy pasta dish gets its rich flavor from the earthy mushrooms, bright dill, and pine nuts, which explode with flavor when toasted.

1 16-ounce package frozen cauliflower florets
12 ounces whole grain penne
1 medium yellow onion, diced small
1 pound sliced cremini or button mushrooms
2 cloves garlic, minced

2 tablespoons chopped fresh dill
1 teaspoon red wine vinegar
sea salt and black pepper to taste
3 tablespoons toasted pine nuts (optional)

1. Bring a large pot of water to a boil. Add the cauliflower and cook until very tender, about 10 minutes.

2. Scoop the cauliflower from the water with a slotted spoon (don't discard the cooking water) and add it to a blender. Puree the cauliflower, adding enough of the cooking water to make a creamy consistency. Set aside the cauliflower puree.

3. Return the pot of water to a boil, salt the water, and add the penne. Cook according to package instructions. Drain the pasta and set it aside.

4. While the pasta cooks, sauté the onion and mushrooms in a large saucepan over medium heat for 8 minutes. Add water 1–2 tablespoons at a time to keep the vegetables from sticking.

5. Add the garlic and dill, and cook for another minute.

6. Add the cauliflower puree, the red wine vinegar, and the cooked pasta.

7. Season with sea salt and black pepper to taste. Serve garnished with the toasted pine nuts.

MAKE IT EASY

You can use light firm silken tofu in place of the cauliflower to save time, but you won't need to boil it. Just add it to the processor, puree until smooth and creamy with the toasted pine nuts, then add it to the cooked mushroom mixture after you add the garlic and dill.

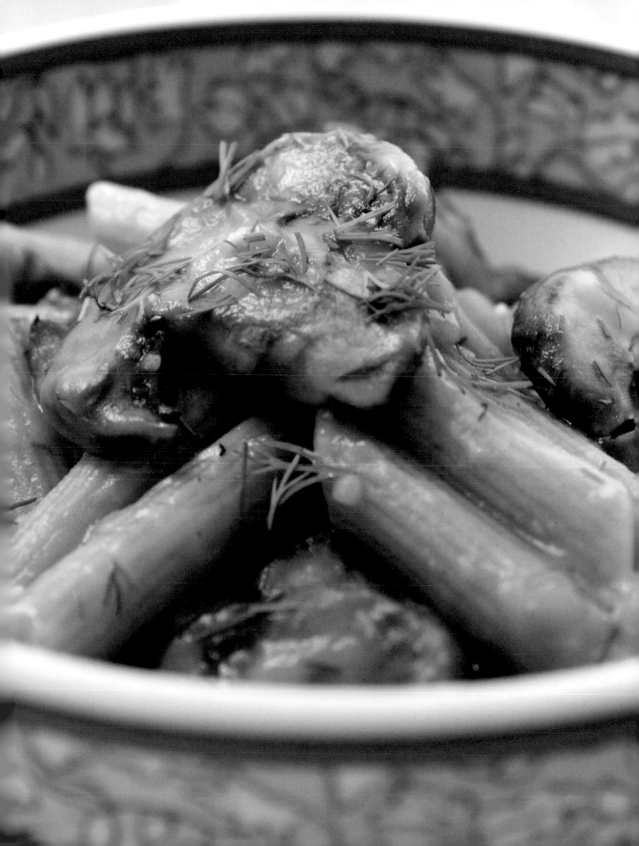

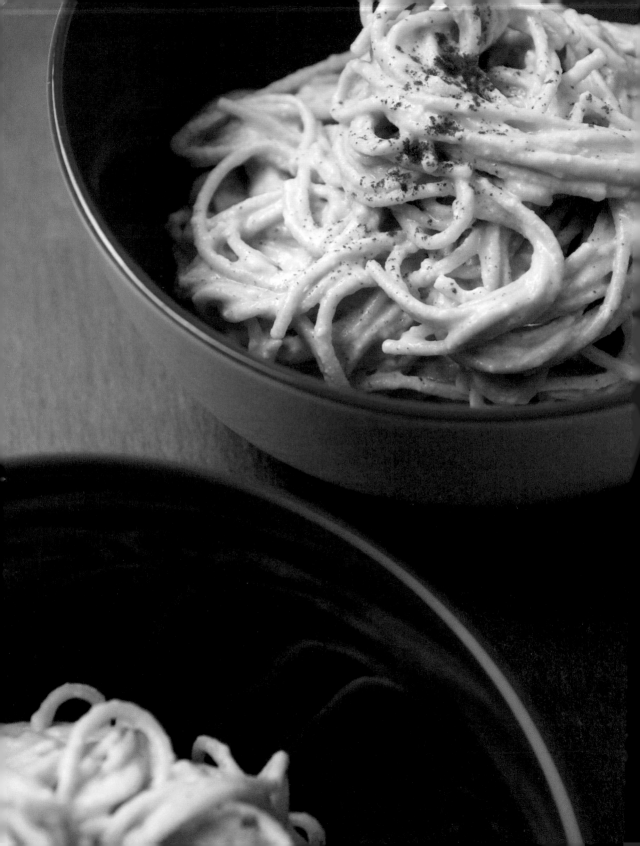

PASTA ALFREDO

MAKES 6 SERVINGS

I used to make traditional Pasta Alfredo for a good friend of mine who proclaimed it "the best ever." Of course we were all addicted to the fat in that recipe. This healthier, whole-grain version is still a treat for me because of the nuts and seeds in the sauce, so I save it for special occasions.

1 pound whole grain fettuccine or linguine
1 cup Alfredo Sauce (p. 68), more or less to taste
sea salt and black pepper to taste

1. Cook the pasta according to package instructions.
2. Drain the pasta and add it to a bowl with the Alfredo sauce. Mix well and taste for sea salt and black pepper.

NO-QUESO MAC AND CHEESE

MAKES 6 SERVINGS

Macaroni and cheese is thought of as the all-American dish. There are as many ways to make it as there are picnics on the Fourth of July. This one has that creamy homemade feel to it with a southwest kick.

12 ounces whole grain macaroni noodles
1 recipe No-Queso Sauce (p. 67)
1 cup nutritional yeast

1. Cook the pasta according to package instructions.
2. Preheat the oven to 375°F.
3. Combine the cooked macaroni noodles, No-Queso Sauce, and nutritional yeast in a large bowl and mix well.
4. Spoon the mixture into a 9 × 13 baking dish and bake for 25 minutes, until the top is lightly browned.

MAKE IT EASY

- For a quicker version, finish heating it on the stovetop for a few minutes instead of baking it.
- If you don't like a spicy mac and cheese, you can cut back on the chipotles in adobo sauce used to make the No-Queso Sauce.

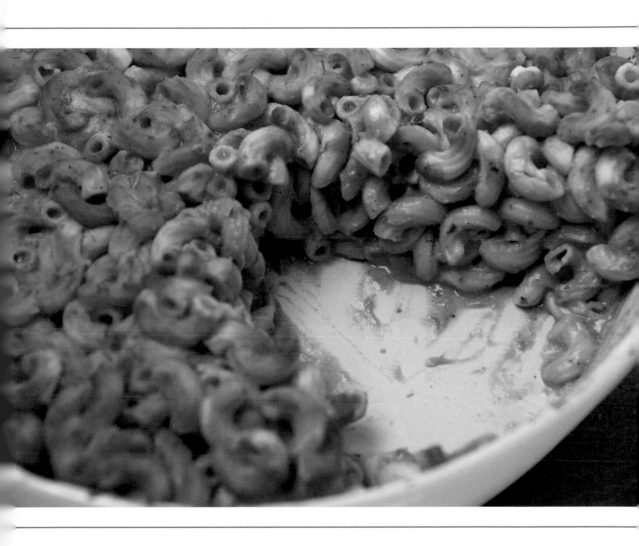

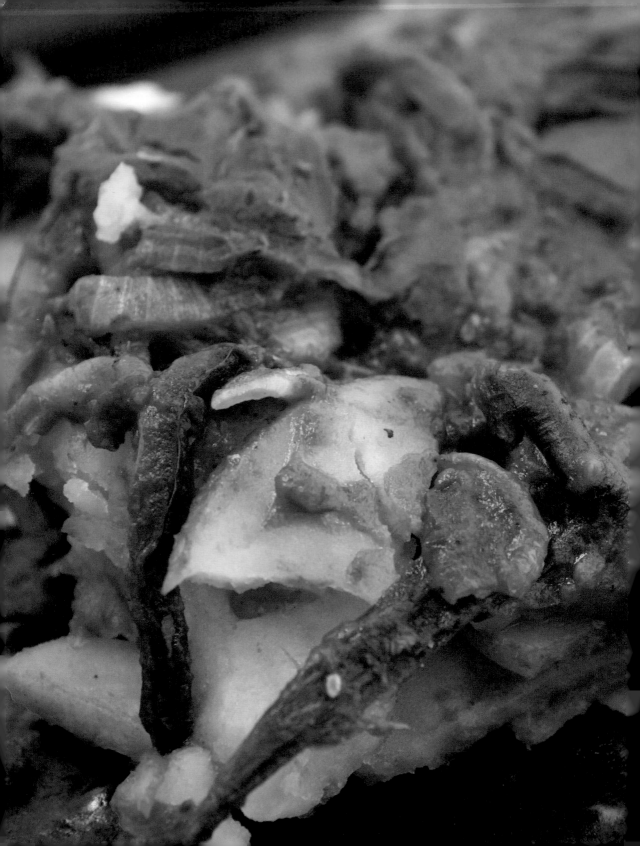

NO-QUESO POTATO BAKE

MAKES 6 SERVINGS

This recipe is one way I like to turn the usual scalloped potatoes into a special dish. When people invite me to a potluck and ask me what I am bringing, I often say scalloped potatoes, then I show up with this dish in hand—much to the delight of the other attendees.

4 large Idaho potatoes, scrubbed and
   thinly sliced
1 large onion, thinly sliced
2 large poblano peppers, seeded and
   thinly sliced

1 recipe No-Queso Sauce (p. 67)
sea salt and black pepper to taste
1 teaspoon paprika

1. Preheat the oven to 425°F.

2. Steam the potatoes for 6 minutes, until tender.

3. While the potatoes steam, sauté the onion and poblano peppers in a large skillet for 6 minutes. Add water 1–2 tablespoons at a time to keep the vegetables from sticking.

4. Add the No-Queso Sauce to the onions and peppers and cook until heated through. Set aside.

5. Spread the steamed potato slices over the bottom of a 9 × 13 baking dish and sprinkle with sea salt and black pepper to taste.

6. Pour the No-Queso Sauce mixture over the potatoes and sprinkle with paprika.

7. Bake for 15 minutes, until bubbly and lightly browned on top. Let cool for 5 minutes before serving.

MAKE IT EASY

- Often I bake several potatoes at the beginning of the week and use them for any number of dishes throughout the week—including this one! If you have extra baked potatoes, you can use them in this dish in place of the steamed potatoes called for in the recipe.
- The poblano peppers have just a little heat and a slightly more peppery flavor than green bell peppers, but you can use bell peppers if you can't find poblanos.

SCALLOPED POTATOES WITH SAFFRON CREAM

MAKES 4–6 SERVINGS

My mom is a great made-from-scratch cook, but my dad had to learn how to cook after my parents divorced in 1967, so many of Dad's early dinners came out of a box. Scalloped potatoes was one of those dishes. This version of one of my favorite comfort foods does not come from a box, but is almost as easy as any boxed version—and much healthier.

3 pounds Yukon gold or red skin potatoes, scrubbed and thinly sliced
2 medium yellow onions, thinly sliced
sea salt and black pepper to taste
1 recipe Saffron Cream (p. 65)

1. Preheat the oven to 425°F.

2. Add the potatoes to a pot with water to cover and cook over medium heat for 5–6 minutes, until the potatoes are just tender. Do not overcook them since they will finish cooking in the oven.

3. While the potatoes cook, sauté the onions over medium heat until they are lightly browned and tender, about 10 minutes.

4. Add half of the potatoes to a 9 × 13 baking dish. Sprinkle with sea salt and black pepper to taste.

5. Pour half of the Saffron Cream over the potatoes. Top with the remaining potatoes, season with sea salt and black pepper again, and spread the rest of the Saffron Cream over the potatoes.

6. Sprinkle the cooked onions over the sauce. Bake for 25 minutes, until bubbly.

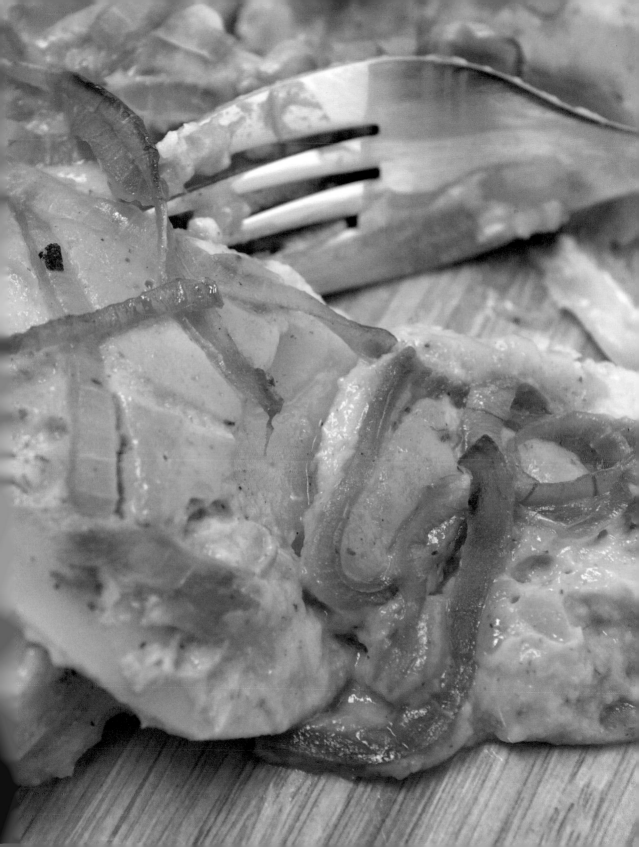

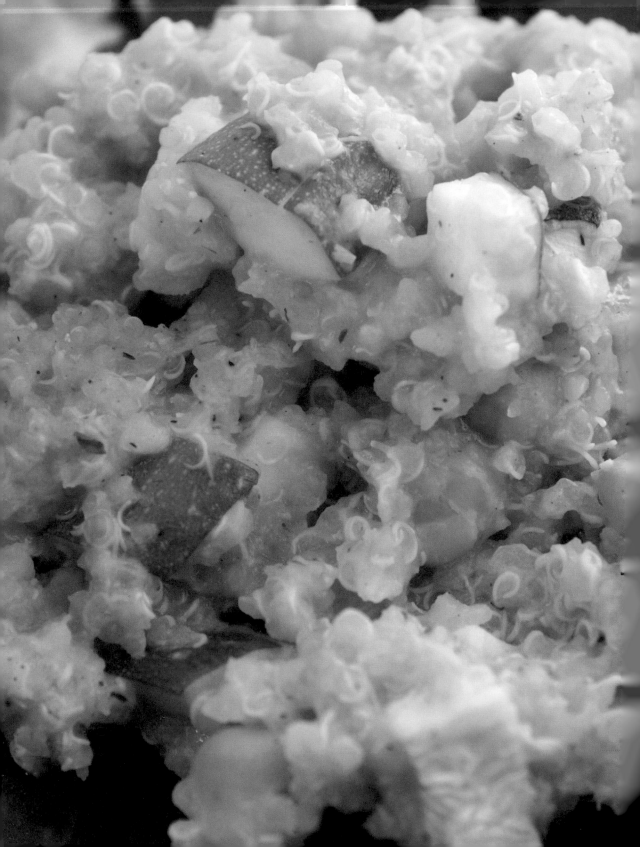

BAKED QUINOA WITH SAFFRON CREAM

MAKES 4 SERVINGS

Think of this dish as an east-meets-west kind of romance. The popular, quick-cooking quinoa from South America meets the classic Mediterranean spice saffron. The two pair nicely in this easy-to-prepare dish, but you could also use cooked brown rice. It's just that quinoa cooks faster. Saffron is the world's most expensive spice, so you might save this dish for a special occasion. Everyone will think you spent all day on it, but I won't tell if you don't.

2 cups water
1 cup quinoa, rinsed
sea salt and black pepper to taste
1 recipe Saffron Cream (p. 65)
1 15-ounce can garbanzo beans (chickpeas), drained and rinsed
1 cup frozen peas
1 large zucchini, diced

1. Preheat the oven to 375°F.
2. Bring the water to a boil and add the quinoa. Reduce the heat to medium, and cook, covered, for 15 minutes, until the quinoa is tender and all the water is absorbed. Season with sea salt and black pepper.
3. Add the cooked quinoa to an 8 × 8 square baking dish with the remaining ingredients. Bake for 20 minutes, until bubbly.

SOUPS

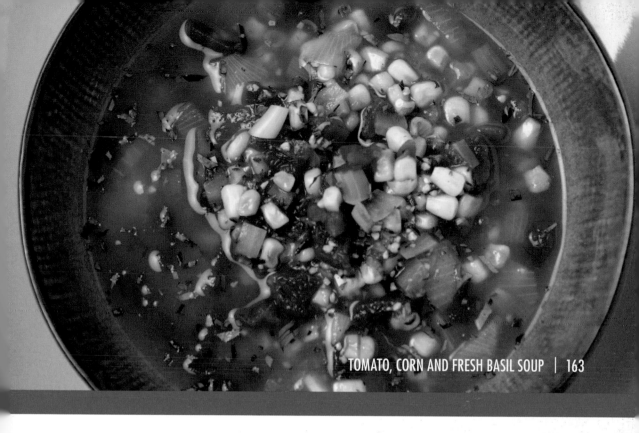

EASY CARROT-GINGER SOUP

MAKES 6 SERVINGS

I am not usually a fan of cooked carrots unless they are part of a rich thick stew or pureed with ginger as in this recipe.

1 small yellow onion, diced
2 celery stalks, diced
5–6 cups vegetable stock
1 tablespoon grated fresh ginger or
   ¾ teaspoon ground ginger
1 tablespoon minced garlic

1 bay leaf
2 10-ounce bags frozen carrots
1 teaspoon sea salt
black pepper to taste
chopped chives for garnish (optional)

1. Combine the onion, celery, 5 cups of the vegetable stock, ginger, garlic, and bay leaf in a large soup pot over medium-high heat and cook for 15 minutes, until the vegetables are tender.

2. Add the frozen carrots and cook for 5 minutes.

3. Season with sea salt and black pepper and cook for another 5 minutes.

4. Remove the bay leaf from the pot, and puree the soup directly in the pot using an immersion blender or in batches with a blender.

5. Add the remaining cup of vegetable stock if the soup is too thick. Taste to add more salt if needed.

6. Serve garnished with the chopped chives.

> **TIP**
>
> If you want to use fresh carrots instead of frozen, you will need about 4 large carrots, peeled and thinly sliced, and cooked with the onion and celery.

TOMATO, CORN, AND FRESH BASIL SOUP PICTURED ON PAGE 161

MAKES 4 SERVINGS

I usually only make this light soup in the summer, mostly because I only use fresh tomatoes when they are perfectly ripe and in season. It comes together quickly so I don't have to heat up the kitchen for a long time, it is light and fresh, and it doesn't slow me down in the summer's heat.

1 medium yellow onion, diced
4 cloves garlic, minced
1 large ripe tomato, diced
2½ cups vegetable stock
3 cups frozen corn
2 teaspoons fresh thyme leaves
1 cup fresh basil leaves, chopped
sea salt and black pepper to taste

1. Sauté the onion in a large saucepan over medium heat for 8 minutes. Add water 1–2 tablespoons at a time as needed to keep the onions from sticking.

2. Add the garlic and cook for another minute.

3. Add the tomato, vegetable stock, frozen corn, and thyme, and cook uncovered for 12 minutes.

4. Add the basil and season with sea salt and black pepper. Remove from the heat.

> **TIP**
>
> For a richer flavor, puree up to half of the soup.

SOUPS **163**

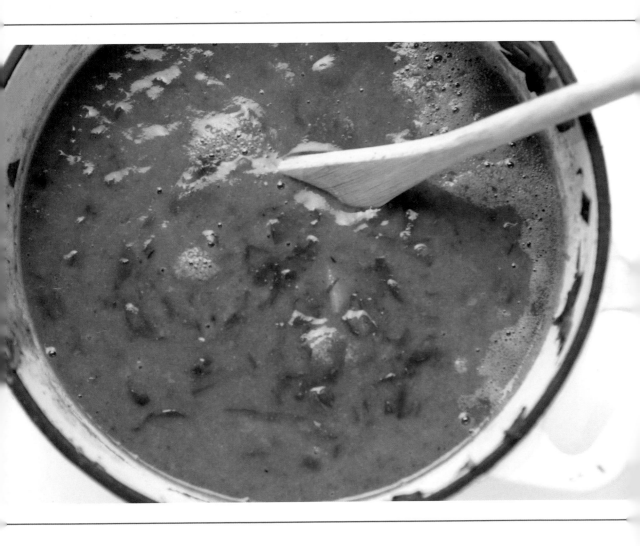

SPINACH-POTATO SOUP

MAKES 4 SERVINGS

I make this soup in the spring with spinach and in the summer and fall with chard or kale. When I use greens other than spinach I don't usually puree it, since I don't like the flavor as much.

1 bunch green onions, sliced
4 cups vegetable stock
3 large Yukon gold potatoes, peeled and diced
2 teaspoons dried thyme
1½ teaspoons ground coriander
6 cups baby spinach, chopped, or
**   1 10-ounce package frozen chopped spinach**
sea salt and black pepper to taste

1. Add the green onions, vegetable stock, potatoes, thyme, and coriander to a large saucepan, and bring to a simmer over medium heat. Cook for 10–12 minutes, until the potatoes are tender.

2. Add the chopped spinach and cook for another 5 minutes, until the spinach has wilted.

3. Puree half the soup in a blender. Return the pureed soup to the pot, season with salt and pepper to taste, and cook for another 5 minutes.

ASIAN NOODLE SOUP

MAKES 4 SERVINGS

The ingredient list for this soup may look long, but the soup comes together quickly and is full of flavor.

4 cups finely sliced Chinese cabbage
10 shiitake mushrooms, stemmed and sliced
1 small red bell pepper, seeded and chopped
6 cups vegetable stock
3 tablespoons low-sodium soy sauce or tamari,
    more or less to taste

2 tablespoons brown rice syrup (optional)
1 tablespoon minced garlic
1 teaspoon ground ginger
4 ounces whole grain noodles
½ cup finely chopped fresh basil or cilantro
1 bunch green onions, sliced

1. Sauté the cabbage, mushrooms, and red bell pepper for 7 minutes in a large stockpot. Add water 1 to 2 tablespoons at a time to keep the vegetables from sticking.

2. Add the vegetable stock, soy sauce or tamari, brown rice syrup, garlic, and ground ginger. Bring the pot to a boil over medium-high heat and cook for 15 minutes.

3. While the vegetable mixture cooks, cook the noodles according to package instructions.

4. Add the basil or cilantro, green onions, and cooked noodles to the stockpot. Simmer for 5 minutes to marry the flavors.

FUSS-FREE PHO

MAKES 4 SERVINGS

This popular Vietnamese noodle soup is full of fresh flavor from herbs added when serving the dish. A lot of effort usually goes into making the broth but not in this version. Star anise and cinnamon give the soup a really unique flavor that complements the fresh herb flavor. If you can find Thai basil, use it.

8 ounces whole grain spaghetti or
    brown rice noodles
6 cups low-sodium vegetable stock
1 3-inch cinnamon stick
1 whole star anise
1 small yellow onion, thinly sliced
4 cloves garlic, minced
1 tablespoon minced fresh ginger

2 heads baby bok choy, thinly sliced
1 cup frozen shelled edamame
2 tablespoons low-sodium soy sauce or tamari
    mung bean sprouts, for garnish
    fresh basil, for garnish
    lime wedges, for garnish
    serrano peppers, thinly sliced, for garnish

1. Cook the noodles according to package instructions. Drain and divide them among four bowls.

2. While the noodles cook, add the vegetable stock, cinnamon stick, star anise, onion, garlic, and ginger to a pot and bring to a boil over high heat. Reduce the heat to medium and simmer the broth for 5 minutes.

3. Add the bok choy, edamame, and soy sauce or tamari and cook for another 8–10 minutes, until the bok choy is tender.

4. Strain the cinnamon stick and star anise from the broth, and ladle the broth and vegetables over the noodles in the serving bowls. Serve the noodle soup with garnishes.

MULLIGATAWNY SOUP

MAKES 4 SERVINGS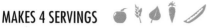

Even if you are not a fan of curry, you will like this soup. The flavor of India's most well-known spice is understated here. Mulligatawny is usually made with fresh apples, but I like the sweetness that ripe pears add to this soup.

1 small yellow onion, diced
2 stalks celery, diced
2 teaspoons toasted curry powder
4 cups vegetable stock
½ cup red lentils
1 12-ounce bag frozen mixed vegetables
2 fresh pears, cored and chopped
1½ cups cooked brown rice
sea salt and pepper to taste

1. Combine the onion, celery, curry powder, vegetable stock, and red lentils in a large saucepan and cook over medium heat for 20 minutes.

2. Add the frozen vegetables and chopped pears, and cook for 10 minutes. Add the cooked brown rice.

3. Season with sea salt and black pepper to taste and cook for 5 minutes more.

> **TIP**
>
> To toast spices, add them to a skillet and turn the heat to medium. Toast, stirring frequently until the spices become fragrant, about 3–4 minutes.

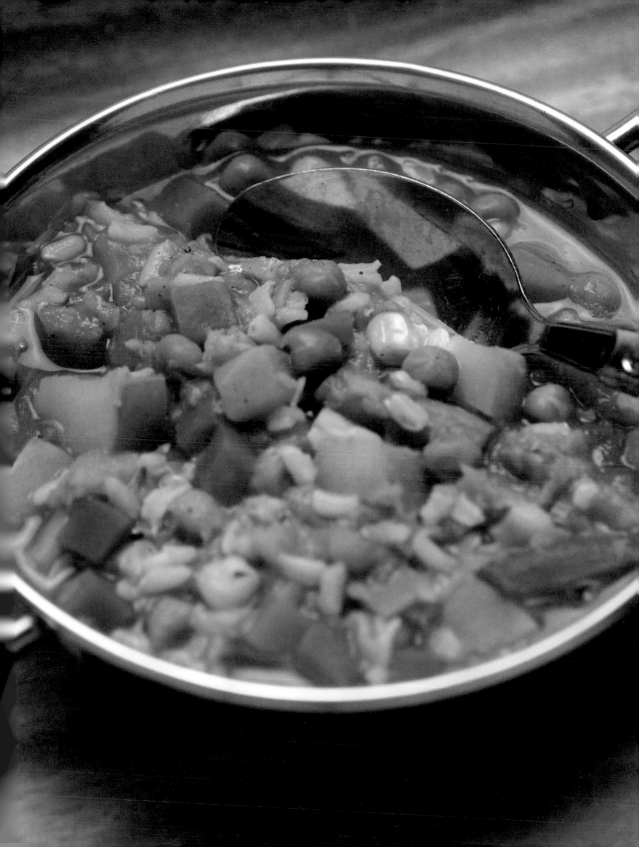

HUNGARIAN MUSHROOM SOUP

MAKES 4 SERVINGS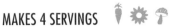

I've had this soup made by one of the best local chefs I know, and even though I don't usually like a "sour" soup, I fell in love with it. The fresh dill makes all the difference in this soup, but dried dill will work in its place. If your dill is old, you may need to add more than 2 tablespoons.

2 large onions, chopped
1½ pounds cremini mushrooms, sliced
2 tablespoons fresh dill, minced
1½ tablespoons paprika

3 cups vegetable stock
2 cups Cauliflower Puree (p. 64)
3 tablespoons red wine vinegar
sea salt and black pepper to taste

1. Sauté the onion and mushroom in a large saucepan for 7–8 minutes, until the onions start to brown. Add water 1–2 tablespoons at a time to keep them from sticking to the pan.

2. Add the dill, paprika, vegetable stock, and Cauliflower Puree, and cook over medium heat for 15 minutes.

3. Add the red wine vinegar and season with salt and pepper to taste.

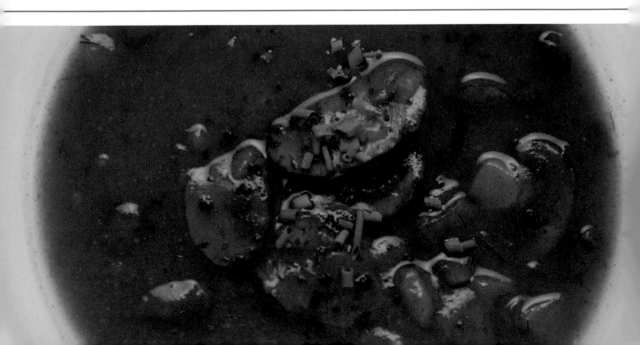

CREAMY POBLANO CORN CHOWDER

MAKES 4 SERVINGS

Chowders are seafood or vegetable stews usually made with milk and often thickened with crackers. This version uses pureed cauliflower as both the milk and the thickener, with flavorful results.

3 cups frozen cauliflower florets
3 cups vegetable stock
1 large yellow onion, diced
2 large poblano peppers, seeded and diced
1½ teaspoons ground cumin

1½ teaspoons dried thyme
1½ teaspoons dried oregano
1 10-ounce bag frozen corn
sea salt and black pepper
chopped fresh cilantro, for garnish

1. Combine the cauliflower and vegetable stock in a 2-quart stockpot and bring the pot to a boil over high heat. Reduce the heat to medium and cook the cauliflower until very tender, about 10 minutes.

2. Add the mixture to a blender with a tight-fitting lid and cover it with a towel. Puree the cauliflower until smooth and creamy, about 3 minutes.

3. While the cauliflower cooks, sauté the onion and poblano peppers in a large saucepan over medium heat for 8 minutes. Add water 1–2 tablespoons at a time to keep the vegetables from sticking.

4. Add the cumin, thyme, and oregano to the onions and peppers, and cook for another minute.

5. Add the corn and the cauliflower puree and cook over medium heat for 15 minutes.

6. Season with sea salt and black pepper and cook for 5 minutes more. Garnish with fresh cilantro.

EASY PEASY BLACK BEAN SOUP

MAKES 4 SERVINGS

You can make this delicious soup without toasting the spices, but it makes all the difference in the flavor. The spices go from toasted to burnt very quickly, so don't leave them unattended.

1 tablespoon ground cumin
2 teaspoons dried oregano
3 cups vegetable stock
1 14.5-ounce can diced tomatoes
3 cloves garlic, minced
3 15-ounce cans black beans, drained and rinsed
sea salt and black pepper to taste
chopped green onion, for garnish
chopped fresh cilantro, for garnish

1. Toast the cumin and oregano in a large saucepan for 3–4 minutes over medium heat, until the spices start to smoke.
2. Add the vegetable stock, tomatoes, garlic, and black beans and cook for 15 minutes.
3. Season with sea salt and black pepper and cook for 5 minutes to marry the flavors.
4. Serve garnished with the green onion and cilantro.

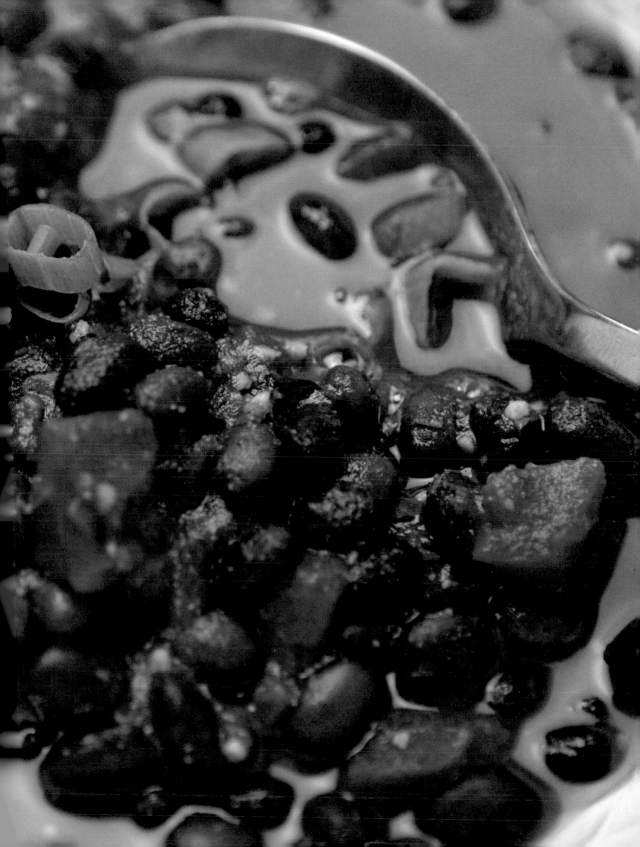

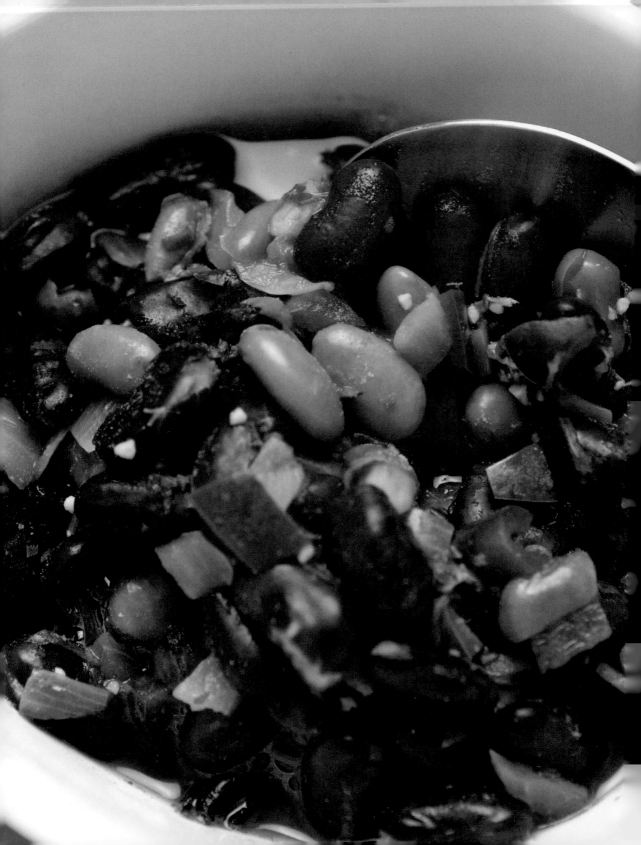

ISLAND RED BEAN STEW

MAKES 6 SERVINGS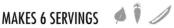

Onions, peppers, garlic, and cilantro cooked with tomato sauce is called *sofrito* and is used commonly in Caribbean cooking to flavor foods. Each household has its favorite version of this flavor starter, and each thinks its own is the best.

1 small yellow onion, finely diced
2 medium poblano peppers, finely diced
4 cloves garlic, minced
½ cup chopped fresh cilantro
4 15-ounce cans red kidney beans (about 7 cups),
   drained and rinsed
½ cup tomato sauce
1 teaspoon dried oregano
sea salt and black pepper to taste
2½ cups vegetable stock

1. Sauté the onion and poblano peppers in a large saucepan over medium-high heat. Cook for 5 minutes, adding water 1–2 tablespoons at a time as needed to keep the vegetables from sticking.

2. Add the garlic and cilantro and cook for 1 minute.

3. Add the red kidney beans, tomato sauce, oregano, sea salt, and black pepper. Mix well.

4. Add the vegetable stock and bring the pot to a boil over high heat. Reduce the heat to medium and simmer, stirring occasionally, for 20 minutes.

SWEET POTATO AND RED PEPPER SOUP

MAKES 6 SERVINGS

The rosemary, nutmeg, and orange zest in this soup really bring the sweet potatoes, leeks, and red pepper to life.

2 large leeks, white and light green parts only, diced and rinsed
1 large red bell pepper, diced
1 teaspoon dried rosemary
¼ teaspoon nutmeg

3 large sweet potatoes, peeled and diced
4 cups vegetable stock
zest of 1 orange
sea salt and black pepper to taste

1. Sauté the leeks and red bell pepper in a large saucepan for 5 minutes. Add water 1–2 tablespoons at a time to keep the vegetables from sticking.

2. Add the rosemary, nutmeg, sweet potatoes, vegetable stock, and orange zest. Bring the pot to a boil over high heat. Reduce the heat to medium and cook the soup until the sweet potatoes are tender, about 12 minutes.

3. Season the soup with salt and pepper and cook for a few minutes more to allow the flavors to marry. Puree up to half the soup for a creamier consistency.

TIP

You can use canned sweet potatoes for this flavorful soup. You will need two 15-ounce cans of sweet potato puree. You can also use pumpkin or other squash in this recipe, but sweet potatoes are my favorite.

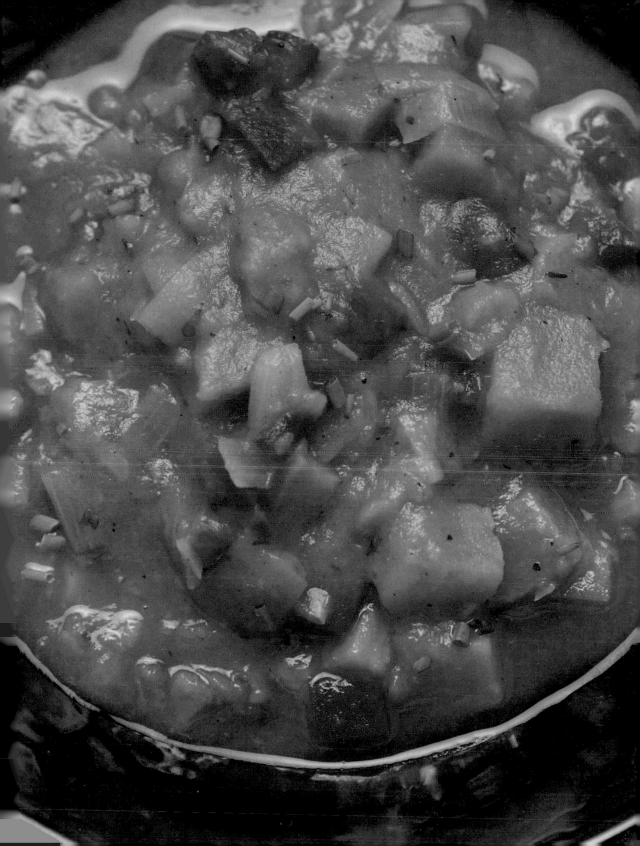

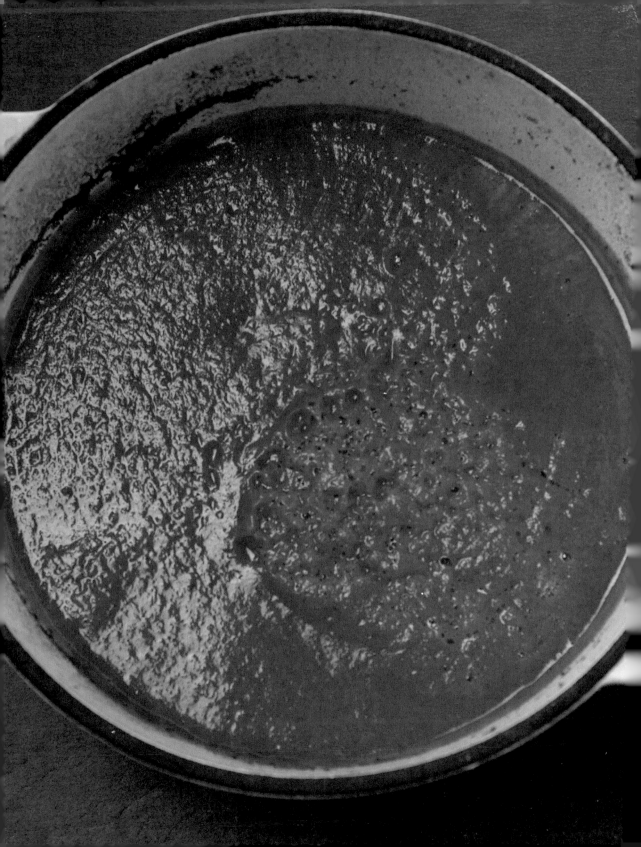

SOUTHWEST TOMATO BISQUE

MAKES 4 SERVINGS

Bisques are cream-based pureed soups made from any number of vegetables. Pureeing vegetables intensifies their flavor. I used to eat bisque like a dip for bread. My mom had to limit me to one or two pieces of bread at a meal because I would eat half a loaf this way.

3–4 cups vegetable stock
2 large tomatoes, diced
1 12-ounce bag frozen cauliflower or
   1 12-ounce package Mori-Nu Silken Lite
   Firm Tofu
4 cloves garlic, minced

2 pitted Medjool dates (optional)
1 tablespoon toasted ground cumin
2 teaspoons toasted dried oregano
2 chipotle peppers in adobo sauce
1 teaspoon sea salt

1. Combine all ingredients in a medium stockpot and cook over medium heat for 10–12 minutes, until the cauliflower is tender.
2. Puree in batches, adding more vegetable stock as needed to make a creamy consistency.

MAKE IT EASY

- Most of the recipes in this book allow you to use silken tofu as a substitute for the cauliflower, especially as a way to save time. If you do so in this recipe, cook everything but the tofu, puree the tofu in a blender until smooth and creamy, and add it to the soup at the very end of cooking before you puree the rest of the soup ingredients.
- To toast ground cumin, add it to a sauté pan over medium-low heat and let it cook until it starts to smell fragrant.
- The dates in this recipe balance out the tartness of the soup very nicely, but they are optional if you like a tangy flavor.

ENTRÉES

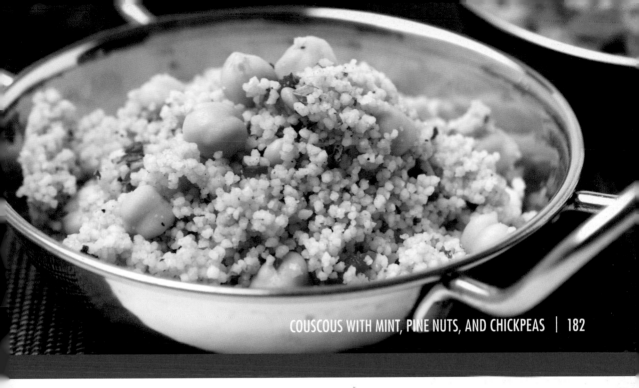

COUSCOUS WITH MINT, PINE NUTS, AND CHICKPEAS PICTURED ON PAGE 181

MAKES 4 SERVINGS

Couscous is a quick-cooking pasta used in a lot of Mediterranean dishes. This is one I eat often when I don't want to spend a lot of time in the kitchen.

3 cups vegetable stock
1½ cups whole grain couscous
2 teaspoons ground coriander
1 15-ounce can garbanzo beans (chickpeas),
   drained and rinsed

¼ cup finely chopped fresh mint
3 tablespoons toasted pine nuts (optional)
zest of 1 lemon
sea salt and black pepper to taste

1. Bring the vegetable stock to a boil in a 2-quart pot with a tight-fitting lid. Add the couscous.

2. Cover with the lid and let sit for 5 minutes, until all the water is absorbed. Add the remaining ingredients, fluff with a fork, and season with sea salt and black pepper to taste.

TIPS

- For a gluten-free version, you could cook 1½ cups of quinoa in 3½ cups of vegetable stock for about 15 minutes, and then continue with the recipe above.
- If you don't like mint, cilantro or basil are both good in its place.

BROCCOLI, RED PEPPER, AND BROWN RICE STIR-FRY

MAKES 2 SERVINGS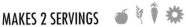

I make a batch of Date and Soy Stir-Fry Sauce once a week so I can make stir-fry whenever I want a quick healthy meal. Sometimes I use fresh vegetables and sometimes I pull a bag of veggies from the freezer. Either way, I've got a healthy meal full of flavor, without a lot of effort.

1 medium yellow onion, thinly sliced
1 medium red bell pepper, thinly sliced
2 cups frozen broccoli florets
¾ cup Date and Soy Stir-Fry Sauce (p. 61)
2 cups cooked brown rice
1 cup mung bean sprouts

1. Heat a large skillet over high heat. Add the onion and red bell pepper and cook for 2–3 minutes, stirring frequently.

2. Add the broccoli and cook for 1 minute, adding water 1–2 tablespoons at a time to keep the vegetables from sticking.

3. Add the stir-fry sauce and cooked brown rice, and cook for 2–3 minutes, until the broccoli is heated through. Add the mung bean sprouts and remove from the heat.

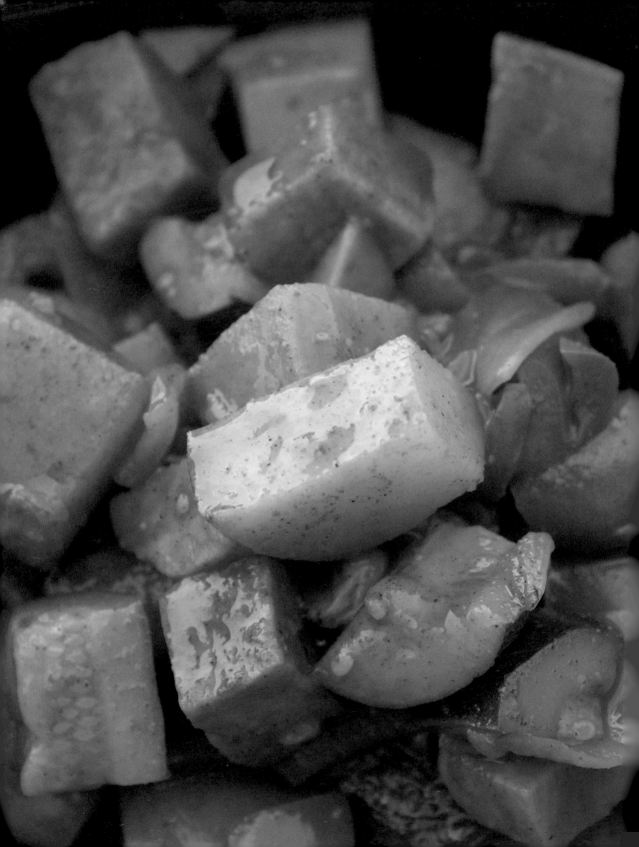

FRUIT AND VEGETABLE CURRY

MAKES 4 SERVINGS

I love the sweet, savory, and pungent flavors in this dish. They all balance each other nicely. The list of ingredients looks long in this curry, but you can make it easier by purchasing frozen chopped onions and peppers. You'll need about 1 cup of each. Serve this over cooked brown rice, quinoa, or your favorite grain.

1 large onion, chopped
1 large sweet potato, peeled and cubed
¼ cup water
2 cups unsweetened apple juice or
    vegetable stock
1 large zucchini, coarsely chopped
1 green bell pepper, chopped

1 large Granny Smith apple, chopped
¼ cup golden raisins
3 cloves garlic, minced
2 teaspoons curry powder
1 teaspoon ground turmeric
1 teaspoon ground cinnamon
sea salt and black pepper to taste

1. Sauté the onion in a large saucepan over medium heat for 5 minutes.
2. Add the sweet potato and water and cook for 5 minutes, until the sweet potatoes are just tender.
3. Add the remaining ingredients and cook for 10 minutes. Season with sea salt and black pepper to taste, and cook for 5 minutes more.

> **TIP**
>
> Ripe pears work well in place of the apples, and feel free to use your favorite dried fruit in place of the raisins (chop larger fruits like apricots).

QUINOA AND WHITE BEANS WITH LEMON AND OLIVES

MAKES 4 SERVINGS

I am still surprised by the number of people I feed at events or in my own home who have never tried quinoa. It is a delicious, nutty grain packed with vitamins and minerals and it's easy to cook. This recipe used to be one of those Mediterranean rice dishes I liked to make until I realized I could get dinner on the table more quickly if I used quinoa instead. So I guess that makes this version a fusion dish (since quinoa is native to South America).

1½ cups quinoa, rinsed
3 cups low-sodium vegetable stock
1 large yellow onion, diced
4 cloves garlic, minced
2 tablespoons dried basil

1 15-ounce can navy beans, drained and rinsed
1 cup pitted kalamata olives, coarsely chopped
juice of 1 lemon
sea salt and black pepper to taste

1. Combine the quinoa and vegetable stock in a medium pot and bring to a boil. Cover with a tight-fitting lid, reduce the heat to medium, and cook the quinoa for 15 minutes until tender.

2. While the quinoa cooks, sauté the onion in a large skillet for 8 minutes. Add water 1–2 tablespoons at a time to keep the onion from sticking.

3. Add the garlic, basil, navy beans, and olives and cook for 5 minutes. Add the cooked quinoa and lemon juice. Season with salt and pepper to taste and cook for 5 minutes more.

POBLANO-CORN QUINOA CAKES

MAKES 4 SERVINGS

Quinoa has a mild nutty flavor and unusual texture, almost like tapioca. It also cooks quickly. These cakes are great for company, especially when you are pressed for time.

¾ cup quinoa, rinsed
1½ cups water
1 medium yellow onion, diced small
1 poblano pepper, diced small
1 teaspoon ground cumin

1 10-ounce package frozen corn
¼ cup arrowroot powder
sea salt and black pepper to taste
1 cup No-Queso Sauce (p. 67) or
   your favorite salsa

1. Add the quinoa to a medium saucepan with the water. Bring the pot to a boil over high heat. Reduce the heat to medium, cover the pot, and cook for 15 minutes or until the quinoa is tender.

2. Preheat the oven to 375°F.

3. While the quinoa cooks, sauté the onion and poblano pepper over medium heat in a skillet for 5 minutes. Add water 1–2 tablespoons at a time to keep the vegetables from sticking.

4. Add the cumin and corn and cook for 2 minutes. Add the cooked quinoa and the arrowroot powder and mix well. Season with salt and pepper to taste.

5. Shape the quinoa mixture into cakes by using a small ice cream scoop or tablespoon and place them on a nonstick baking sheet or one lined with parchment paper. Gently flatten the cakes until they are ½-inch thick.

6. Bake the cakes for 20 minutes. Serve with No-Queso Sauce or salsa.

JERK-STYLE BEANS

MAKES 4 SERVINGS

I make these beans whenever I want a change from the usual baked beans I see at every summer picnic. I love black-eyed peas any way you make them, but use whatever beans you have on hand to make this dish.

1 medium yellow onion, diced
1 red bell pepper, diced
1 15-ounce can tomato sauce
2 teaspoons Jerk Spice Rub (p. 57), more to taste
2 15-ounce cans black-eyed peas, drained and rinsed
sea salt to taste

1. Sauté the onion and red bell pepper in a saucepan over medium heat for 5 minutes, until the onion starts to brown. Add water 1–2 tablespoons at a time as needed to keep the vegetables from sticking.

2. Add the tomato sauce, Jerk Spice Rub, and black-eyed peas. Simmer for 15 minutes. Season with sea salt and cook for a few minutes more.

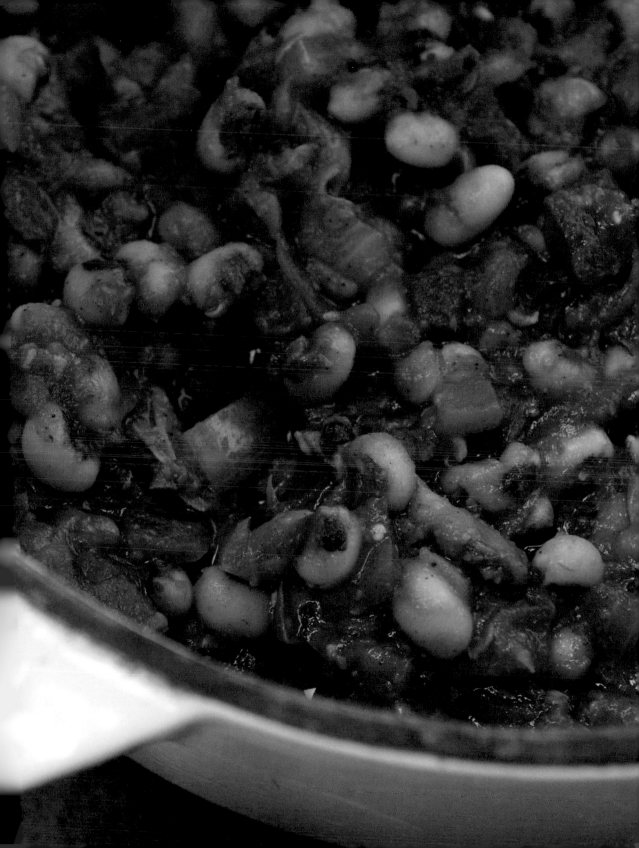

POLENTA ROUNDS WITH SAFFRON CREAM AND WILTED SPINACH

MAKES 4 SERVINGS

You can buy precooked polenta in the natural foods section of your grocery store or you can make Easy Creamy Polenta. Polenta, like most grains, adapts well to any number of flavors, even saffron. If you prefer, you can use arugula instead of the spinach.

1 18-ounce package precooked polenta or
   1 recipe Easy Creamy Polenta (p. 36), set in muffin tins
1½ pounds fresh baby spinach
sea salt and black pepper to taste
1 recipe Saffron Cream (p. 65), warmed

1. Slice the polenta into ¾-inch-thick rounds. Place them in a nonstick skillet and warm over medium-low heat for about 3 minutes. Flip and warm the other side for 3 minutes.

2. Remove the polenta rounds from the skillet and set them aside. Add the spinach to the skillet with a little water and salt and pepper. You may need to add the spinach in batches.

3. Cook until the spinach wilts, about 5 minutes. Divide it among four plates and top with the polenta rounds. Serve topped with the Saffron Cream.

ZUCCHINI, CORN, AND RED PEPPER PANCAKES

MAKES 4 SERVINGS

I eat these pancakes often in the summer when zucchini and basil flourish in the garden. And while you can serve them with a dollop of your favorite plant-based sour cream, I usually eat them as they are, with a salad or brown rice. They are creamy all on their own and don't need much help in the flavor department.

2 medium zucchini
6 green onions, thinly sliced
1½ cups corn, fresh or frozen
½ large red bell pepper, finely diced

½ cup fresh basil leaves, finely chopped
½ cup whole wheat pastry flour
1 teaspoon baking powder
sea salt and black pepper to taste

1. Grate the zucchini on the large holes of a box grater. Place the grated zucchini in a bowl with the remaining ingredients and mix well.

2. Heat a nonstick skillet over medium heat.

3. Drop ½-cup measures of the zucchini mixture onto the heated skillet. Cook them for 4 minutes without touching them. Gently turn them over and cook the other side for 3 minutes.

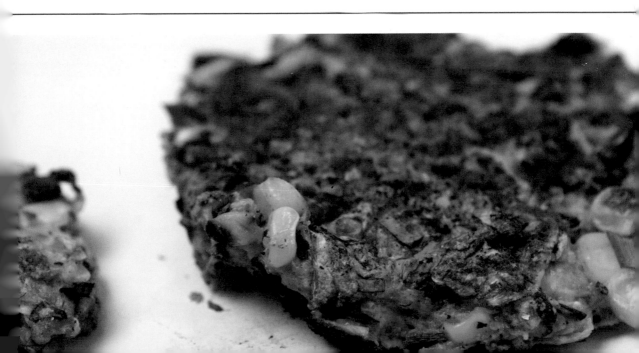

MEDITERRANEAN VEGETABLE STEW

MAKES 4 SERVINGS

Cinnamon, coriander, and saffron are classic flavors in parts of the Mediterranean. And while a lot of stews can take hours to prepare, this one takes less than 30 minutes and doesn't sacrifice any of that great flavor. Serve this over couscous, brown rice, or whatever grain you have on hand.

1 medium yellow onion, diced
1 large red bell pepper, cut into ¾-inch cubes
2 cups vegetable stock
1 16-ounce package frozen vegetables (look for a large, chunky vegetable blend)
1 15-ounce can garbanzo beans (chickpeas), drained and rinsed

1 15-ounce can tomato sauce
1 teaspoon ground cinnamon
1 teaspoon ground coriander
1 generous pinch saffron
sea salt and black pepper to taste
chopped fresh cilantro, for garnish

1. Sauté the onion and red bell pepper for 5 minutes. Add water 1–2 tablespoons at a time to keep the vegetables from sticking.

2. Add the remaining ingredients (through saffron) and cook, covered, over medium heat for 12 minutes.

3. Season with sea salt and black pepper to taste and cook for another 5 minutes. Serve garnished with the chopped cilantro.

EGGPLANT-TOMATO-OLIVE RAGU

MAKES 4 SERVINGS

Sometimes I take leftovers and throw them into a pot and see what happens. This is one of my favorite results. I wanted to make an eggplant stir-fry one day and thought I had stir-fry sauce made. Turns out I didn't, but I did have hummus, and the rest is history. The Basil Pesto Hummus is a perfect complement to the eggplant, tomato, and olives. It is creamy but not too rich. Eat this with cooked grains or tossed with your favorite whole-grain pasta.

1 large yellow onion, diced
1 large eggplant, cut into 1-inch cubes (about 7–8 cups)
1 large tomato, diced
1 cup pitted kalamata olives
1 cup Basil Pesto Hummus (p. 73)

1. Sauté the onion and eggplant for 8 minutes over medium heat. Add water 1–2 tablespoons at a time to keep the vegetables from sticking.

2. Add the tomato and olives and cook for 5 minutes more.

3. Add the Basil Pesto Hummus and cook for 5 minutes until bubbly.

> **TIP**
>
> Saffron Cream (p. 65) is a great alternative to the hummus for a change.

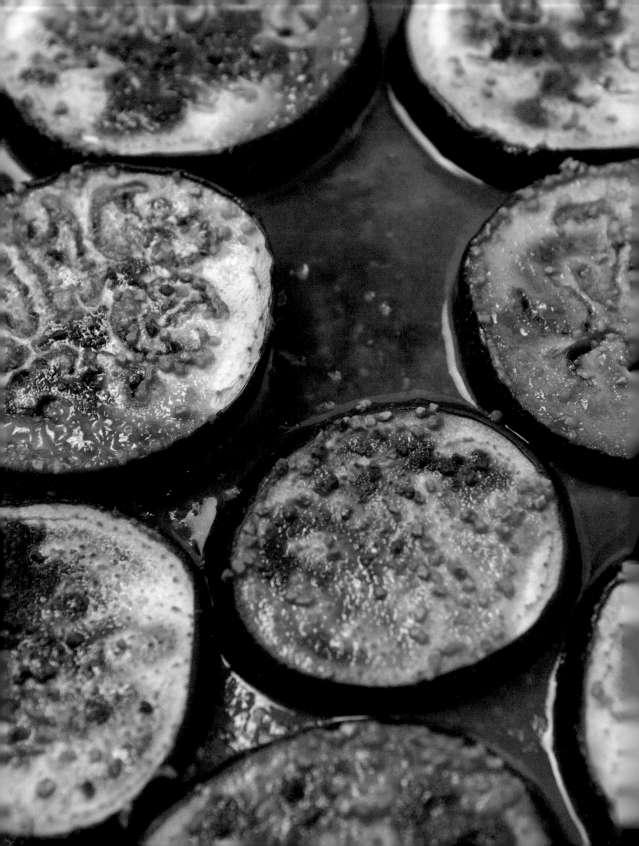

GLAZED EGGPLANT CUTLETS

MAKES 4–6 SERVINGS

Serve this as a sandwich with Red Pepper Slaw (p. 113) or Peanut Slaw (p. 114), or serve it over cooked brown rice or quinoa with steamed vegetables.

1 large eggplant, cut into ½-inch slices
¼ cup low-sodium soy sauce or tamari
¼ cup Two-Minute Date Puree (p. 62) or maple syrup
2 tablespoons Dijon mustard
¼ teaspoon cayenne pepper (optional)

1. Preheat the oven to 375°F. Place the eggplant slices on a nonstick baking dish or one lined with parchment paper.
2. Combine the remaining ingredients in a small bowl and whisk to mix well.
3. Pour the tamari mixture over the eggplant slices. Bake the eggplant for 20 minutes.

MUSHROOMS BARBACOA

MAKES 4 SERVINGS

Barbacoa is a form of slow-cooking meat over an open fire that supposedly originated in the Caribbean (although humans have been cooking this way since we discovered fire). The term "barbecue" is actually derived from *barbacoa* and both have become very popular foodie trends. I use a spice blend popular in the *barbacoa* style to make this quicker-cooking mushroom recipe. Serve this easy flavorful dish over brown rice or quinoa for a simple meal or use it to flavor Mushroom Tacos (p. 206) or Barbacoa Mushroom Burritos (p. 123).

4 cloves garlic
1 medium yellow onion, coarsely chopped,
   divided
3 tablespoons lime juice
2–3 chipotle peppers in adobo sauce
1 tablespoon ground cumin

1 tablespoon ground oregano
pinch ground cloves
2 pounds portobello mushrooms, cut into
   ½-inch cubes
sea salt and black pepper to taste

1. Combine the garlic, half of the onion, and the lime juice, chipotle peppers, cumin, oregano, and cloves in a blender and process until smooth. Set aside.

2. Heat a large skillet over medium-high heat. Add the remaining onion and the mushrooms, and cook, stirring frequently, until the mushrooms have released their juices and cooked down, about 10 minutes.

3. Season with sea salt and black pepper to taste. Add the marinade and reduce the heat to medium. Cook for 10 minutes, until the sauce has thickened.

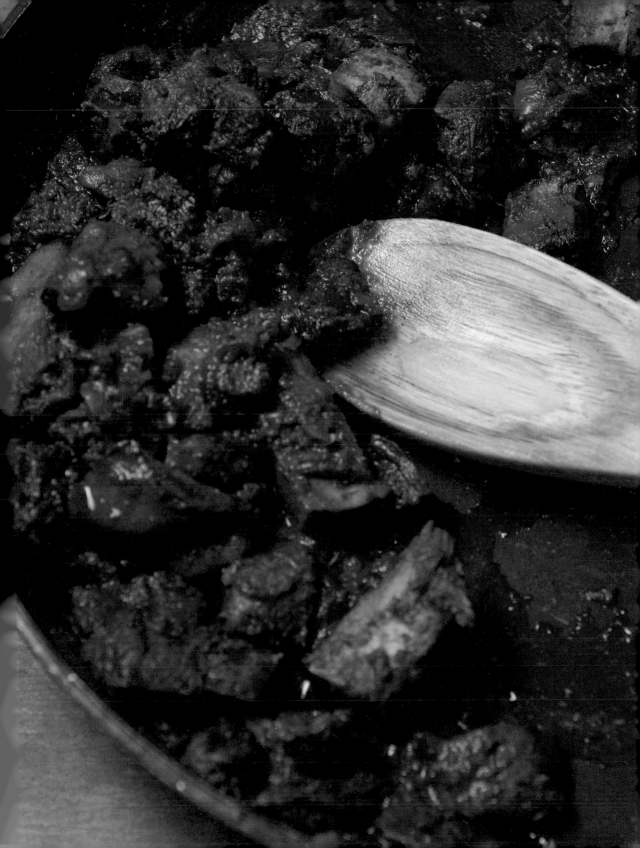

JERK MUSHROOMS

MAKES 4 SERVINGS

I sometimes leave these mushrooms whole and make a burger out of them, but often I cube them so I can eat them with rice or stick them in a wrap. The rub for this dish is not as spicy as traditional jerk rubs, so if you like it hotter, add more cayenne pepper.

2 pounds portobello mushrooms, cubed
1 large yellow onion, chopped
sea salt and black pepper to taste
4 tablespoons Jerk Spice Rub (p. 57), more or less to taste

1. Heat a large skillet over medium-high heat. Add the mushrooms and onion and cook, stirring frequently, until the mushrooms have released their juices and cooked down, about 10 minutes.

2. Season with sea salt and black pepper to taste. Add the jerk rub and reduce the heat to medium. Cook for 10 minutes.

BURRITO BOWL

MAKES 4 SERVINGS

Many of my favorite meals include rice and veggies. I always have both on hand so that a quick and healthy meal is not far away. I make several variations of this bowl and some kind of well-seasoned mushroom is often on the menu. They are versatile, flavorful, and satisfying.

4 cups cooked brown rice or other grain, divided
1 recipe Mushrooms Barbacoa (p. 196) or Jerk Mushrooms (p. 198)
1 avocado, diced
½ medium red onion, diced
2 ripe Roma tomatoes, chopped
½ cup chopped fresh cilantro
1 lime, quartered

1. Place 1 cup of cooked rice in the bottom of each of four bowls.
2. Top each bowl with the mushrooms and a little of each of the avocado, red onion, tomatoes, and chopped cilantro.
3. Serve each bowl with one of the lime quarters.

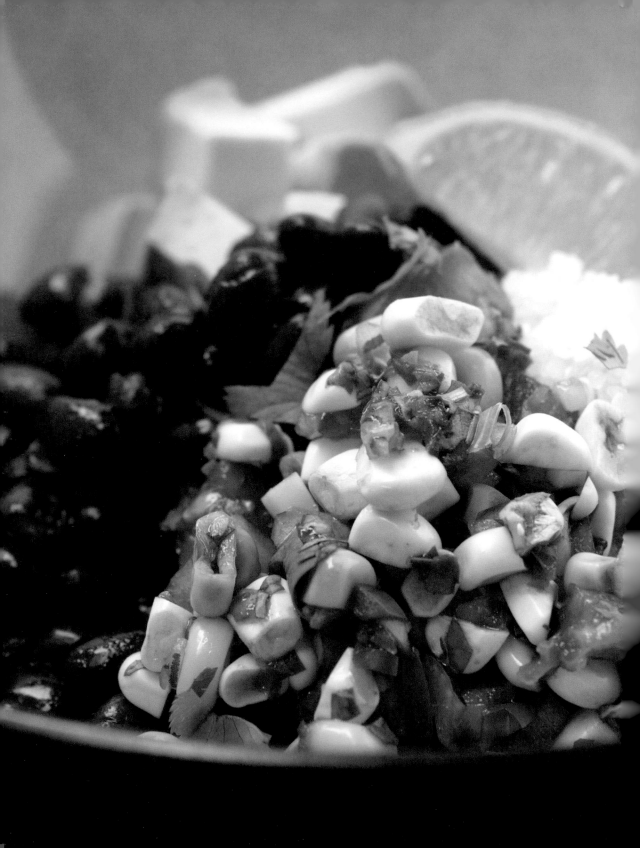

QUINOA–BLACK BEAN BUDDHA BOWL

MAKES 4 SERVINGS

I make some kind of Buddha bowl or Zen bowl a few times weekly. I like them because it is not always about making a pretty presentation—sometimes you just want to get the food on the table. I make a big pot of some grain—quinoa is my favorite because of its nutty flavor and quick cooking time—once a week to have on hand, add some kind of sauce or salsa like the one in this recipe, and use frozen vegetables if I am in a hurry (fresh steamed vegetables when I have a little more time).

3 cups water
1½ cups quinoa, rinsed
1 teaspoon sea salt
2 15-ounce cans black beans, drained and rinsed
1 recipe Fresh Herbed Tomato-Corn Salsa (p. 58)
1 ripe avocado, cubed
½ cup chopped fresh cilantro

1. Bring the water to a boil in a medium pot. Add the quinoa and salt. Bring the pot back to a boil over high heat, reduce the heat to medium, and cook the quinoa, covered, for 15 minutes, until tender.

2. Add the black beans and cook just until heated.

3. Divide the quinoa–black bean mixture among four bowls and top with the salsa, avocado, and chopped cilantro.

FALAFEL BOWL

MAKES 4 SERVINGS

This is one of my favorite bowls. I usually make a double batch of the falafel so I can use half of it in Falafel Tacos (p. 205) or Mediterranean Pita Pizzas (p. 211), too. This recipe is probably my favorite way to eat falafel because it means I get a good serving of vegetables for dinner.

4 cups cooked brown rice
1 package frozen mixed vegetables,
   cooked according to package instructions
1 recipe Falafel (p. 82)
1 cup Green Sauce (p. 52)
chopped green onion or cilantro, for garnish

1. Put 1 cup of cooked brown rice in the bottom of each of the four bowls.

2. Top each bowl with some of the cooked vegetables, Falafel, and Green Sauce.

3. Garnish with chopped green onion, cilantro, or both.

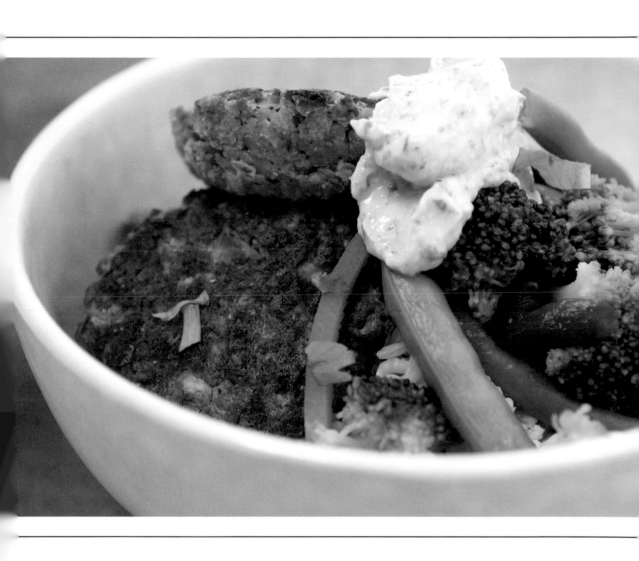

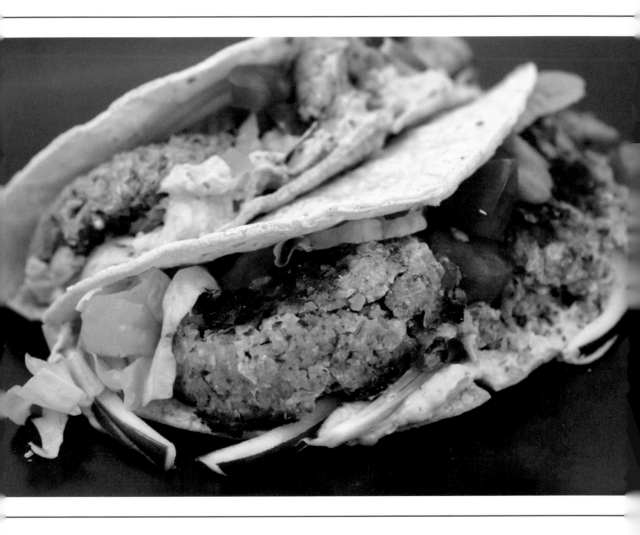

FALAFEL TACOS

MAKES 4 SERVINGS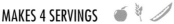

One day I made falafel for a few friends and realized right before the first guest arrived that I had forgotten to buy pita bread. One of my guests said that she often serves falafel in corn tortillas, either with Green Sauce or with salsa, and voilà, dinner was saved!

12–16 6-inch corn tortillas
1 recipe Falafel (p. 82)
1 cup Green Sauce (p. 52) or
your favorite salsa, more as desired
2 cups chopped romaine lettuce
1 large tomato, chopped
1 medium red onion, diced

1. Preheat a nonstick skillet over medium heat for 5 minutes. Add enough corn tortillas to cover the bottom of the pan and heat for 3–4 minutes to soften the tortillas. Repeat with the remaining tortillas.
2. To serve, cut each falafel in half and place two or three halves in the center of each corn tortilla.
3. Top each tortilla with some of the Green Sauce, romaine lettuce, tomato, and red onion.

MUSHROOM TACOS

MAKES 4 SERVINGS

I eat tacos more than a few times monthly. They are easy, versatile, and full of flavor. I like this version because of how quickly it comes together. I make extra batches of all of the components—the Mushrooms Barbacoa, the Peanut Slaw, and even the Asian Salad Dressing (p. 45), used to make the slaw—and use them in a variety of ways throughout the week.

12–16 6-inch corn tortillas
1 recipe Mushrooms Barbacoa (p. 196)
1 recipe Peanut Slaw (p. 114)
chopped fresh cilantro, for garnish
fresh lime wedges, for garnish

1. Preheat a large nonstick skillet over medium heat for 5 minutes.
2. Add enough corn tortillas to cover the bottom of the pan in a single layer and heat for 3–4 minutes. Repeat with the remaining tortillas.
3. To serve: place slices of the Mushrooms Barbacoa in the center of each tortilla and spoon some of the slaw on top. Garnish with the chopped cilantro and serve with the lime wedges as a garnish.

TOSTADAS

MAKES 4 SERVINGS

I think of tostadas like open-face tacos. Like with tacos, you can use whatever filling you like. In this recipe, the refried beans are filling, the Fresh Herbed Tomato-Corn Salsa adds a fresh flavor to the dish, and the avocados add extra creaminess.

12 6-inch corn tortillas
1 15-ounce can fat-free refried beans
1 recipe Fresh Herbed Tomato-Corn Salsa (p. 58)
1 ripe avocado, diced small

1. Heat the corn tortillas a few at a time in a nonstick skillet over medium heat until they start to brown, about 5 to 6 minutes.

2. Place the tortillas on a work surface and spread 2–3 tablespoons of refried beans over each tortilla. Top with ¼ cup of the salsa and some of the diced avocado.

CAULIFLOWER PARMESAN

MAKES 4 SERVINGS

This unusual take on a popular Italian dish is one of my favorite comfort food dishes. It has all of the flavors of the original without all of the fat and dairy. This dish takes a little more effort than most in this cookbook, so save it for guests or for when you want to treat yourself to something special. Steam the leftover cauliflower and use it in the Quinoa–Black Bean Buddha Bowl (p. 201), or on a salad.

2 heads cauliflower
½ cup water
sea salt and black pepper to taste
12 ounces whole grain linguine
6 cloves garlic

1 tablespoon dried basil
1 teaspoon dried oregano
6–8 tablespoons Del's Favorite
   Parmesan (p. 56)
1½ cups pasta sauce

1. Turn the oven on to broil and heat to 425°F.

2. Bring a large pot of water to a boil.

3. Cut the cauliflower heads in half through the stem, then trim each half so you have a cutlet 1–1½ inches thick.

4. Place the cauliflower cutlets in a large skillet and add the ½ cup water to the pan. Cook the cutlets for 5 minutes over medium heat, until almost tender. Season with sea salt and black pepper to taste and place the cutlets on a nonstick baking sheet or one lined with parchment paper.

5. Cook the pasta in the boiling water according to package instructions.

6. Add the garlic, basil, and oregano to a blender and puree for 30 seconds. Drizzle the garlic mixture evenly over the cooked cauliflower cutlets and sprinkle Del's Favorite Parmesan on top.

7. Bake the cutlets for 8–10 minutes, until the cutlets are lightly browned.

8. To serve, divide the cooked linguine among four plates and top with the pasta sauce. Place a cauliflower cutlet on top of the pasta sauce for each plate.

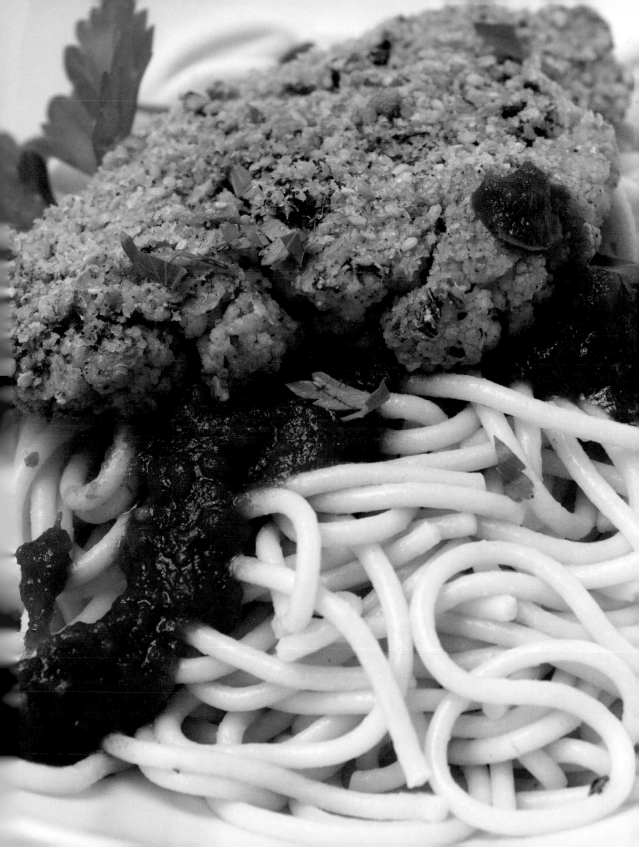

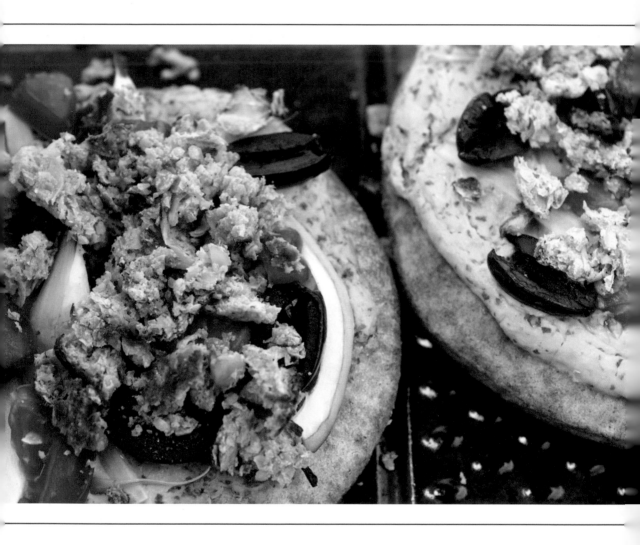

MEDITERRANEAN PITA PIZZA

MAKES 4 SERVINGS

Pizza was always a special event in our house. Mom and Dad usually cooked most of our meals, so it always felt like a holiday when we ordered pizza from our favorite pizzeria. I still eat pizza on occasion, but I don't make traditional cheese- and meat-laden ones. And when I'm in a hurry, I prefer a ready-made crust, but oil-free, whole grain versions are hard to find. So I make pita pizzas. They do the job as nicely as the large traditional crusts, and each person gets his or her own individual pizza. The other nice part about pita pizzas is that you can more easily customize each pizza.

4 6-inch whole grain pitas
1 recipe Green Sauce (p. 52)
1 recipe Falafel (p. 82), cooked according to instructions, then crumbled

1 small red onion, thinly sliced
1 cup sliced black olives
1 cup chopped fresh cilantro

1. Preheat the oven to 350°F.
2. Place each pita on a flat surface and top with ½ cup of the Green Sauce.
3. Sprinkle the crumbled falafel on top of the sauce and top with the red onion and sliced olives.
4. Bake the pita pizzas for 12–15 minutes. Serve garnished with the chopped cilantro.

VARIATION — THAI PITA PIZZA

Replace the Green Sauce with Almost Instant Peanut Sauce (p. 51). Top with sliced red onion and Mushrooms Barbacoa (p. 196), and serve garnished with chopped fresh cilantro.

PITA PIZZA ALFREDO

MAKES 4 SERVINGS

Here's another one of my favorite pita pizzas based upon a pizza *bianca* I used to order from a local pizzeria. The olives, artichoke hearts, and fresh basil are classic Mediterranean foods and give the pizzas a burst of flavor on top of the already flavorful Alfredo sauce.

4 6-inch whole grain pitas
1 cup Alfredo Sauce (p. 68)
1 small red onion, diced
1 cup canned artichoke hearts, quartered
½ cup kalamata olives, pitted and halved
1 cup chopped fresh basil

1. Preheat the oven to 350°F.
2. Place each pita on a baking sheet and top with ¼ cup of the Alfredo sauce.
3. Top with the red onion, artichoke hearts, and sliced olives.
4. Bake the pita pizzas for 12–15 minutes. Serve garnished with the chopped basil.

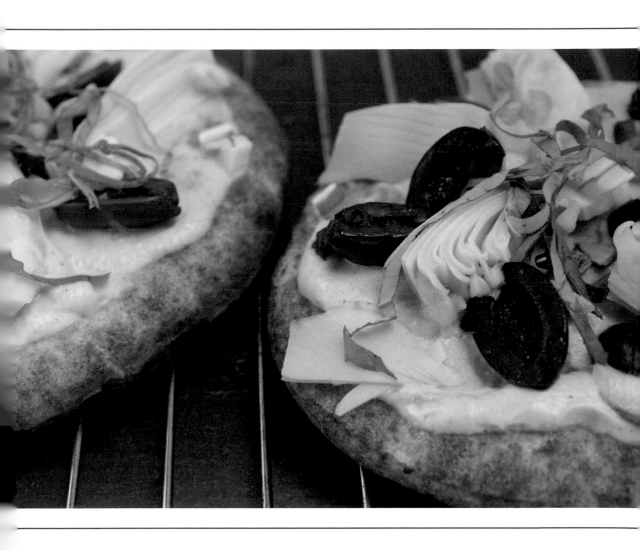

DESSERTS

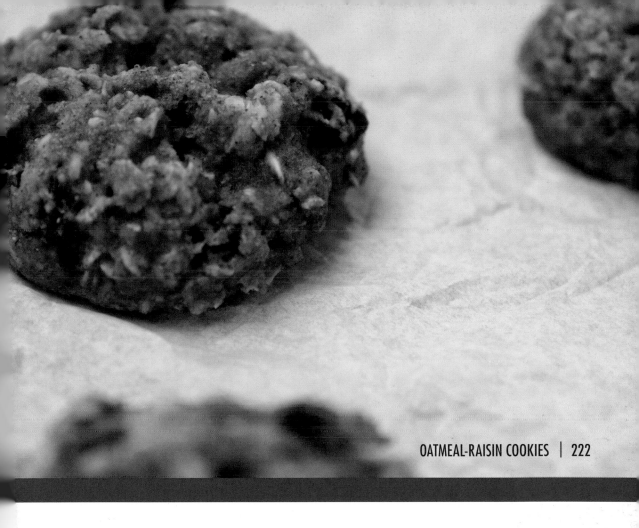

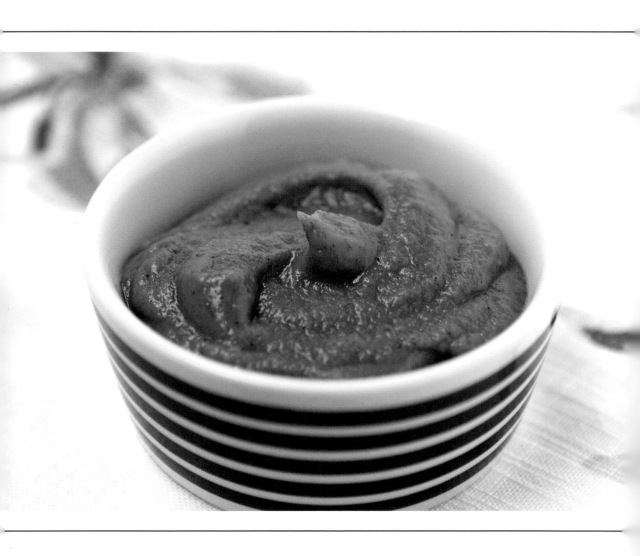

ALMOST INSTANT SWEET POTATO PUDDING

MAKES 4 SERVINGS

Sweet potato pie is one of my favorite desserts. But the fattening crust and the sugar-laden filling always left my stomach feeling heavy. This pudding makes me forget all about that indulgent pie while giving me the creamy flavor I love. And, even better, I don't have to turn on the oven.

2 15-ounce cans mashed or pureed sweet
    potatoes (about 3 cups)
¾ cup Two-Minute Date Puree (p. 62) or
    ½ cup maple syrup
2 tablespoons almond butter (optional)
2 teaspoons vanilla extract

½ teaspoon ground cinnamon
½ teaspoon ground allspice
¼ teaspoon sea salt
zest of 1 orange
½ cup unsweetened nondairy milk

1. Put all of the ingredients except the nondairy milk in a food processor. Puree until smooth, adding the nondairy milk until the desired consistency is achieved.

2. Serve immediately or refrigerate for 1 hour before serving.

MAKE IT EASY

- If you can't find canned sweet potato puree, you can use canned pumpkin.
- The almond butter is optional, but it really does make the pudding creamier, so make this dessert when you can have it as a treat.

STOVETOP FRUIT CRISP

MAKES 4 SERVINGS

I never make fruit crisp in the summer if it means I have to heat up the whole house by turning on the oven. With this version, I don't have to. I use apples in this recipe, but you can use fresh ripe pears or peaches for a nice change.

TOPPING

1 cup rolled oats
¾ cup Two-Minute Date Puree (p. 62) or
　½ cup maple syrup
1 teaspoon ground cinnamon
pinch sea salt

FILLING

3 cups chopped apples (I like Granny Smith)
¾ cup Two-Minute Date Puree (p. 62) or
　½ cup maple syrup
1 teaspoon ground cinnamon
pinch nutmeg
pinch sea salt

1. To make the topping, add the oats to a medium saucepan and toast over medium-low heat for 5 minutes until they are fragrant and start to brown. Add the Two-Minute Date Puree or maple syrup, cinnamon, and sea salt. Cook for 5 minutes, until the oats have absorbed most of the syrup. Set aside.

2. To make the filling, combine the apples, Two-Minute Date Puree or maple syrup, cinnamon, nutmeg, and sea salt in a saucepan and cook over medium heat until the apples soften, about 6 minutes.

3. To assemble, spoon the filling mixture into individual serving bowls and sprinkle the oat mixture over it.

BANANA-COCONUT MACAROONS

MAKES 14–16 MACAROONS

I love the flavor of bananas and coconut together, and they make an unusual but delicious macaroon. Coconut is a high-fat food, so these are definitely a treat.

⅓ cup Two-Minute Date Puree (p. 62) or
   ½ cup maple syrup
1 ripe banana, coarsely chopped
¼ cup water
2 cups unsweetened shredded coconut
¼ cup whole wheat pastry flour
1 teaspoon vanilla extract
pinch sea salt (optional)

1. Preheat the oven to 350°F.
2. Combine the Two-Minute Date Puree or maple syrup and the banana in the bowl of a food processor. Puree until smooth.
3. Add the remaining ingredients and process until well combined.
4. Using a small ice cream scoop or tablespoon, shape the dough into balls and place on a nonstick or silicone-lined baking sheet.
5. Bake for 12–13 minutes, until lightly browned. Let cool completely and store refrigerated in an airtight container for up to 7 days.

GERMAN CHOCOLATE NO-BAKE COOKIES

MAKES 10–12 COOKIES

These cookies are inspired by my love for German chocolate cake, German chocolate cookies, or German chocolate anything! Toasting the pecans and the coconut really brings out their flavor.

½ cup pecans
¾ cup unsweetened shredded coconut
1 cup Medjool dates, pitted
1 tablespoon unsweetened cocoa

1. Toast the pecans and shredded coconut in a 350°F oven for 5 minutes.
2. Add the toasted mixture to the bowl of a food processor with the remaining ingredients and process until the mixture starts to form a ball.
3. Using a small ice cream scoop or tablespoon, shape the dough into cookies and place on a baking sheet.
4. Refrigerate for 1 hour until set. Store in an airtight container for up to 7 days.

PEAR AND FIG COOKIES

MAKES ABOUT 12 LARGE COOKIES

These soft cookies are one of my favorite cookies that don't have chocolate in them. I grew up loving Fig Newtons and it was thirty years before I ate figs in any other dish.

1½ cups whole wheat pastry flour
1 cup finely chopped figs
1½ teaspoons baking powder
¼ teaspoon ground nutmeg

½ cup maple syrup or ⅓ cup Two-Minute
   Date Puree (p. 62)
½ cup unsweetened applesauce
1 large ripe pear, grated
pinch sea salt (optional)

1. Preheat the oven to 350°F.
2. Combine the flour, chopped figs, baking powder, and nutmeg in a mixing bowl and whisk to combine.
3. Make a well in the center of the flour mixture, add the remaining ingredients, and fold together.
4. Using a small ice cream scoop or tablespoon, drop the dough onto a parchment-lined, silicone-lined, or nonstick baking sheet.
5. Bake the cookies for 10 minutes, until they start to brown and don't give when gently pressed on the top.
6. Let the cookies cool on the baking sheet for 5 minutes before moving to a wire rack to cool completely.

TIPS

- Use fresh figs if you can find them, but I usually have dried figs on hand.
- You can also use apples instead of pears, or use any other dried fruit you have available.

OATMEAL-RAISIN COOKIES

MAKES 12 LARGE OR 24 SMALL COOKIES

I have always and will always love cookies. Oatmeal-raisin cookies were the first dessert I learned how to make, following the recipe off of the Quaker Oats box when I was less than ten years old. Of course, the cookies I made back then were filled with sugar, white flour, and margarine. Try these instead!

2 cups oats
1½ cups whole wheat pastry flour
1 cup raisins
1½ teaspoon baking powder
1 teaspoon ground cinnamon

pinch sea salt
¾ cup maple syrup or 1¼ cups Two-Minute
  Date Puree (p. 62)
1 cup unsweetened applesauce
½ teaspoon vanilla extract

1. Preheat the oven to 350°F.

2. Combine the oats, flour, raisins, baking powder, cinnamon, and sea salt in a large bowl and mix well.

3. Make a well in the center of the flour mixture and add the remaining ingredients. Gently fold together.

4. Using a small ice cream scoop or tablespoon, shape the cookies into balls and place them on a parchment-lined, silicone-lined, or nonstick baking sheet.

5. Bake large cookies for about 15 minutes. Bake small cookies for about 12 minutes. The cookies should be lightly browned on top.

6. Let the cookies cool on the baking sheet for 10 minutes before moving them to a wire rack to cool completely.

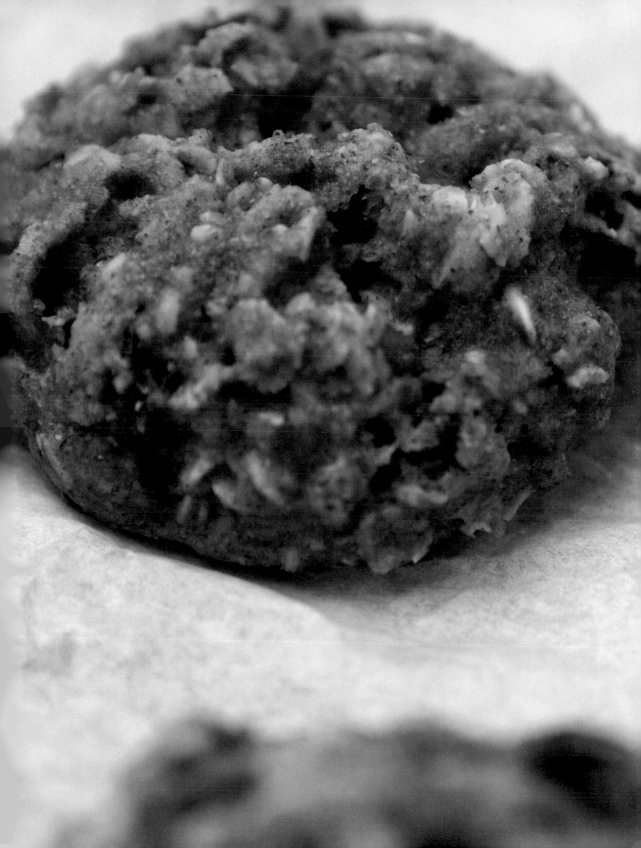

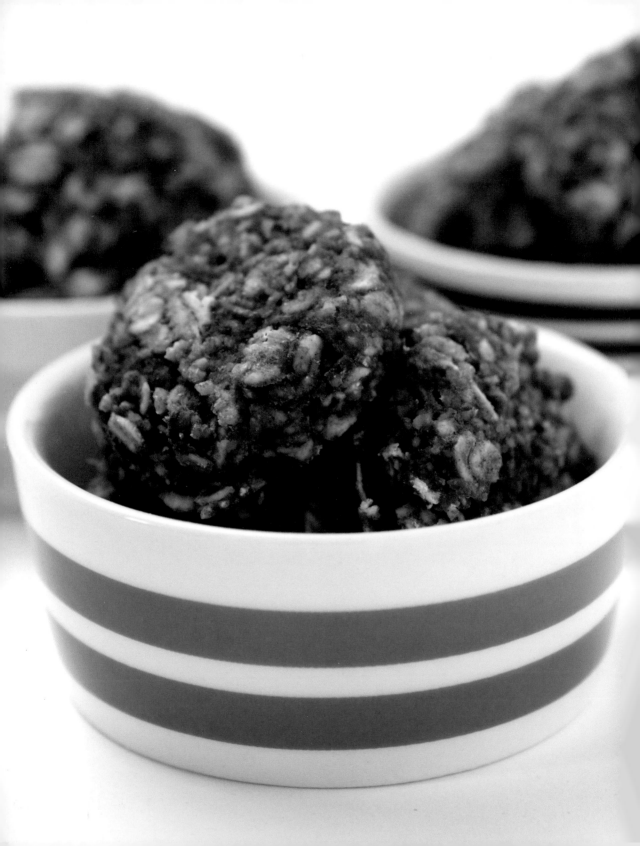

BANANA–PEANUT BUTTER COOKIES

MAKES 10 LARGE OR 20 SMALL COOKIES

I used to make a smoothie called Chunky Monkey with bananas, peanut butter, and cocoa. It is one of my favorite flavor combinations, so I use it here in this recipe—and even without the cocoa, these cookies make me grin from ear to ear.

10 Medjool dates, pitted
1 ripe banana (overripe is fine)
½ cup peanut butter
¼ cup unsweetened applesauce

1 teaspoon vanilla extract
2½ cups quick-cooking or rolled oats
¼ cup whole wheat pastry flour
¼ teaspoon baking powder

1. Preheat the oven to 350°F.
2. Add the dates to a small pan with enough water to cover and cook for 5 minutes over medium heat. Then puree the mixture in a food processor until smooth and creamy.
3. Add the banana, peanut butter, applesauce, and vanilla to the food processor and puree until smooth and creamy.
4. Transfer the peanut butter–banana mixture to a bowl and add the remaining ingredients, stirring until just combined.
5. Using a small ice cream scoop or tablespoon, drop spoonfuls of dough onto a parchment-lined, silicone-lined, or nonstick baking sheet.
6. Bake large cookies for about 15 minutes. Bake small cookies for about 12 minutes. The cookies should be lightly browned on top.
7. Let the cookies sit for about 10 minutes before removing them from the baking sheet; they will be easier to remove. Move the cookies to a wire rack to cool completely.

PINEAPPLE POPS

MAKES 10–12 ICE POPS

These ice pops don't really qualify as quick, but they sure are easy—and tasty too. If you want to use fresh pineapple, you will need to peel and core it. Make sure to find good, ripe fruit.

2 15-ounce cans unsweetened pineapple,
   drained, reserving the juice

1. Place the pineapple in a blender and process until mostly smooth. Add enough of the reserved juice to make a creamy consistency.

2. Spoon the pineapple into ice pop molds, add wooden sticks, and freeze until solid, about 1 hour.

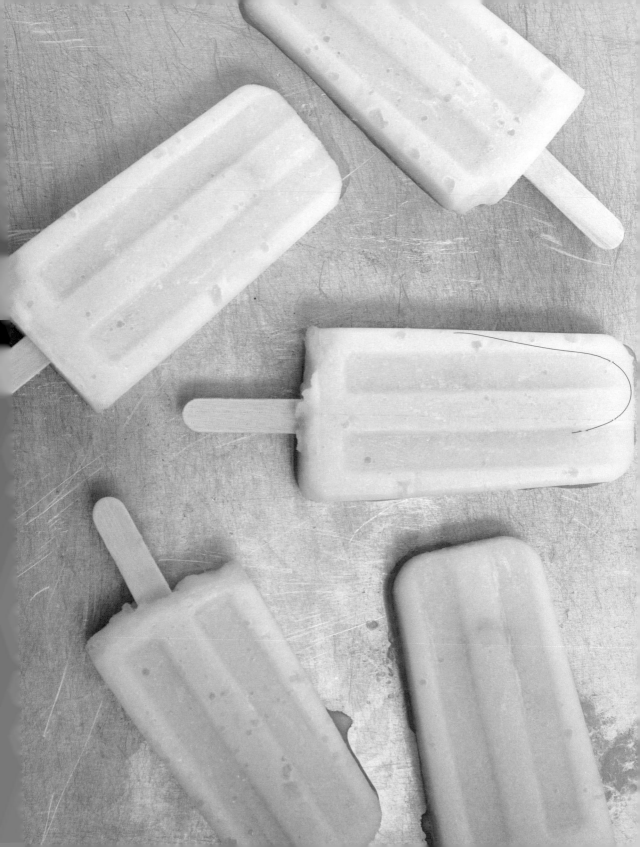

RED BEAN ICE POPS

MAKES 8 ICE POPS

I have eaten ice pops for as long as I can remember. I am one of those kids who went running through the house, screaming, to ask my mom for money when I heard the ice cream truck coming down the street. This recipe is my healthy version of a Fudgsicle. Think of all that fiber you get every time you eat one—and without a lick of added processed sugar.

1 15-ounce can adzuki beans, drained and rinsed
1¼ cups light coconut milk
1 cup Medjool dates, pitted
3 tablespoons unsweetened cocoa
½ teaspoon vanilla extract
pinch sea salt

1. Combine all ingredients in a blender and process until smooth and creamy.
2. Use a spatula or wooden spoon to scrape the mixture down into the bottom of the blender jar to make sure everything is processed.
3. Pour the mixture into ice pop molds and place a wooden stick in each mold.
4. Freeze until solid, about 1 hour, before serving.

VARIATION — CHUNKY MONKEY ICE POPS

Add 3 tablespoons of peanut butter to the blender with all of the other ingredients and mix well.

APPENDIX

MEASUREMENT GUIDE

ABBREVIATION KEY

tsp   =   teaspoon
tbsp   =   tablespoon
dsp   =   dessert spoon

U.S. STANDARD — U.K.

¼ tsp   =   ¼ tsp (scant)
½ tsp   =   ½ tsp (scant)
¾ tsp   =   ½ tsp (rounded)
1 tsp   =   ¾ tsp (slightly rounded)
1 tbsp   =   2½ tsp
¼ cup   =   ¼ cup minus 1 dsp
⅓ cup   =   ¼ cup plus 1 tsp
½ cup   =   ⅓ cup plus 2 dsp
⅔ cup   =   ½ cup plus 1 tbsp
¾ cup   =   ½ cup plus 2 tbsp
1 cup   =   ¾ cup plus 2 dsp

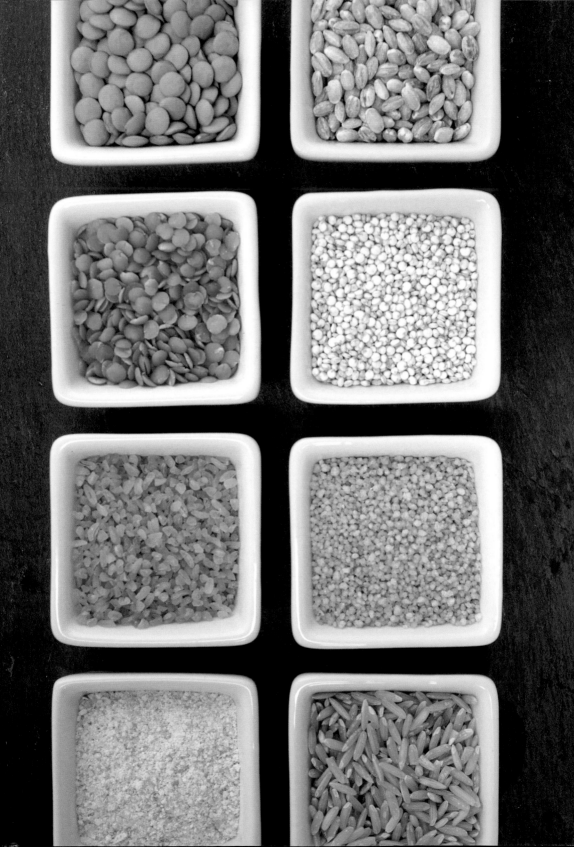

DIETARY SYMBOLS

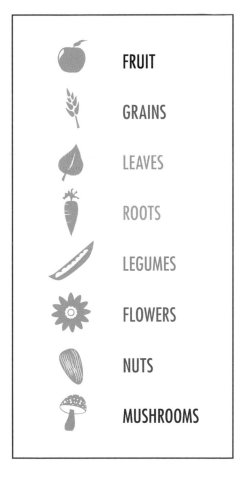

FRUIT

GRAINS

LEAVES

ROOTS

LEGUMES

FLOWERS

NUTS

MUSHROOMS

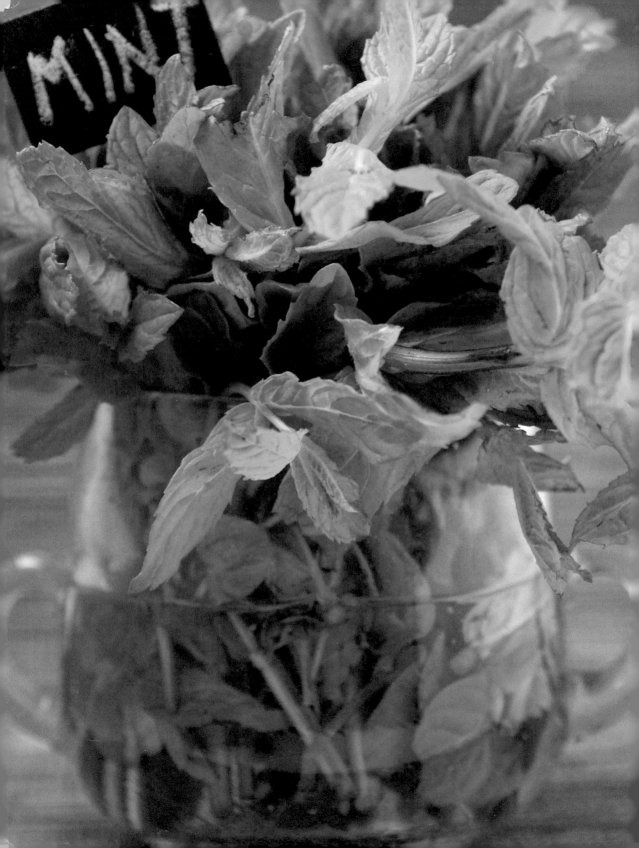

NUTRITIONAL VALUE

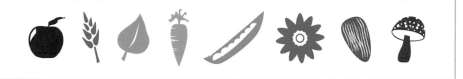

Here's a look at some of the nutritional value of the eight categories (seven types of plant parts plus mushrooms):

FRUITS are packed with vitamin C and other phytochemicals.

GRAINS abound in carbohydrates, fiber, minerals, and B vitamins.

LEAVES are lush with antioxidant vitamins, fiber, and complex carbohydrates.

ROOTS have lots of carbohydrates; some have carotenoids.

LEGUMES are a hearty source of protein, fiber, and iron.

FLOWERS are rich in antioxidants and phytochemicals.

NUTS are loaded with omega-3 fats, vitamin E, and protein.

MUSHROOMS offer a good supply of selenium and other antioxidants.

To be consistent with the message in *The China Study* and especially its sequel, *Whole*, nutrient compositions are not presented with the recipes. Nutrient contents in different samples of the same food often are highly variable, leading consumers to be concerned with trivial and meaningless differences instead of the far more important health characteristics of food variety and wholesomeness.

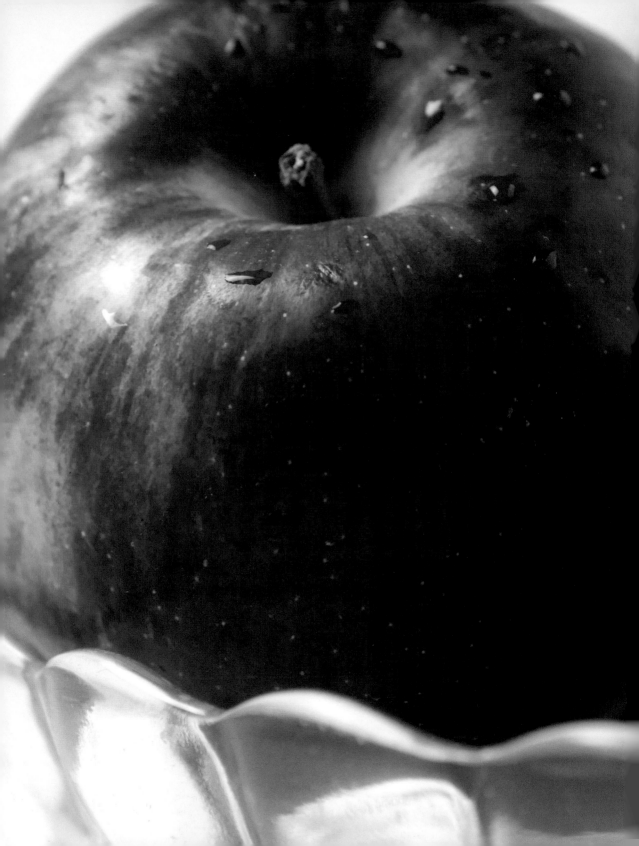

INDEX

ABOUT THE AUTHOR

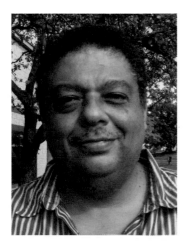

Del Sroufe has worked in vegan and vegetarian kitchens for more than twenty-three years, most recently as chef and co-owner of Wellness Forum Foods, a plant-based meal delivery and catering service that emphasizes healthy, minimally processed foods. He teaches cooking classes and is the author of *Better Than Vegan* and *Forks Over Knives: The Cookbook*. He has also contributed recipes to *Food Over Medicine* by Dr. Pam Popper and Glen Merzer.

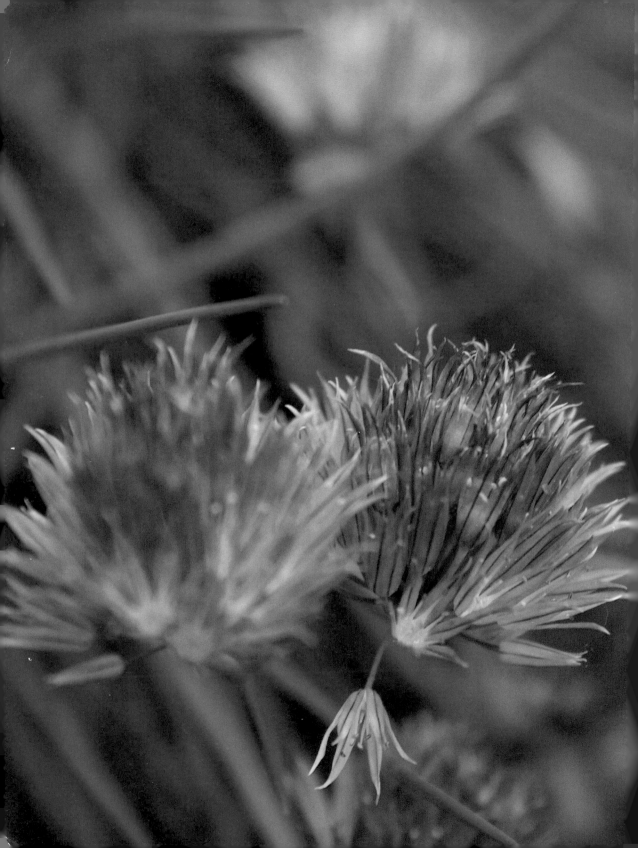

ABOUT THE EDITOR

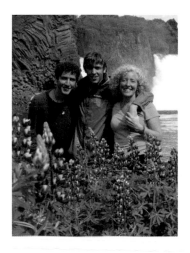

LeAnne Campbell, PhD, who lives in Durham, North Carolina, has been preparing meals based on a whole food, plant-based diet for almost twenty years. LeAnne has raised two sons—Steven and Nelson, now twenty-one and twenty years of age—on this diet. As a working mother, she has found ways to prepare quick and easy meals without using animal products or adding fat. She is the *New York Times* best-selling author of *The China Study Cookbook*, published by BenBella Books in 2013, and editor of *The China Study All-Star Collection* (2014). She is currently the founder and executive director of the Global Leadership Institute, an education program focused on community, culture, and change, and Atravesando Fronteras, an environmental justice program providing conferences and training, located in the Dominican Republic.

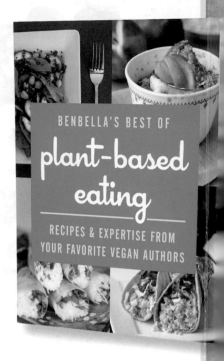
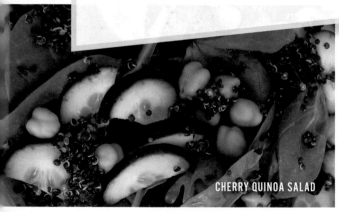

CHERRY QUINOA SALAD

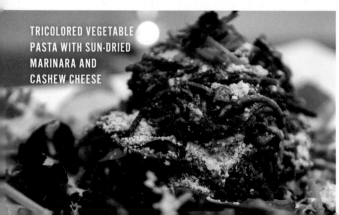

TRICOLORED VEGETABLE PASTA WITH SUN-DRIED MARINARA AND CASHEW CHEESE

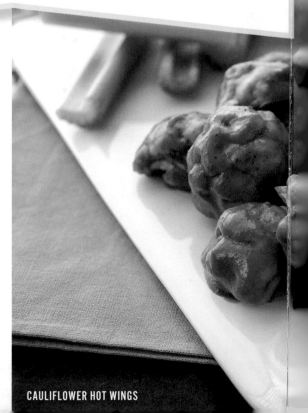

CAULIFLOWER HOT WINGS